Pearls of Wisdom on How I Did It

by
Addie L. Robinson

authorHOUSE™

1663 LIBERTY DRIVE, SUITE 200
BLOOMINGTON, INDIANA 47403
(800) 839-8640
WWW.AUTHORHOUSE.COM

First published by AuthorHouse 09/14/05

ISBN: 1-4208-5989-7 (sc)

Library of Congress Control Number: 2005904708

Printed in the United States of America
Bloomington, Indiana

This book is printed on acid-free paper.

Contact:
P.O Box 6530
Philadalphia, P.A. 19138
www.addierobinson.com

Before

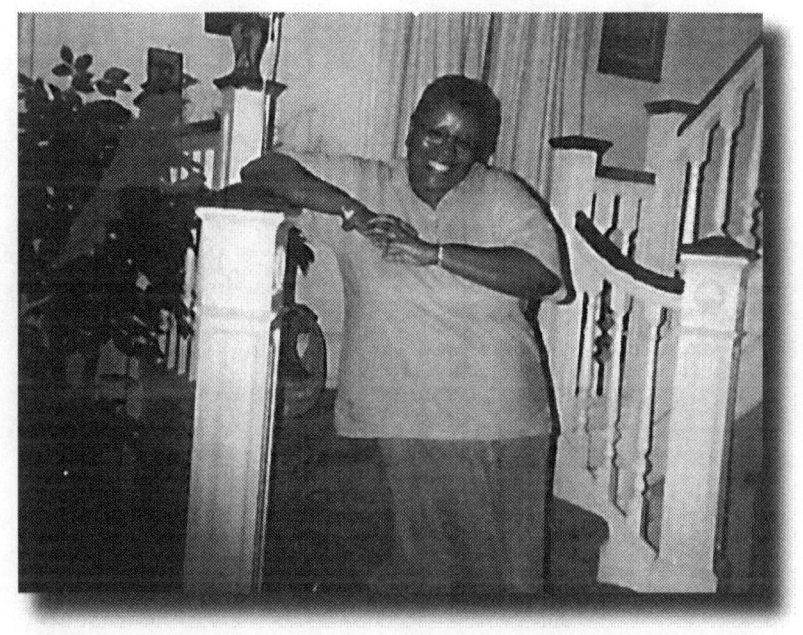

Addie L. Robinson
At
Size 22

During

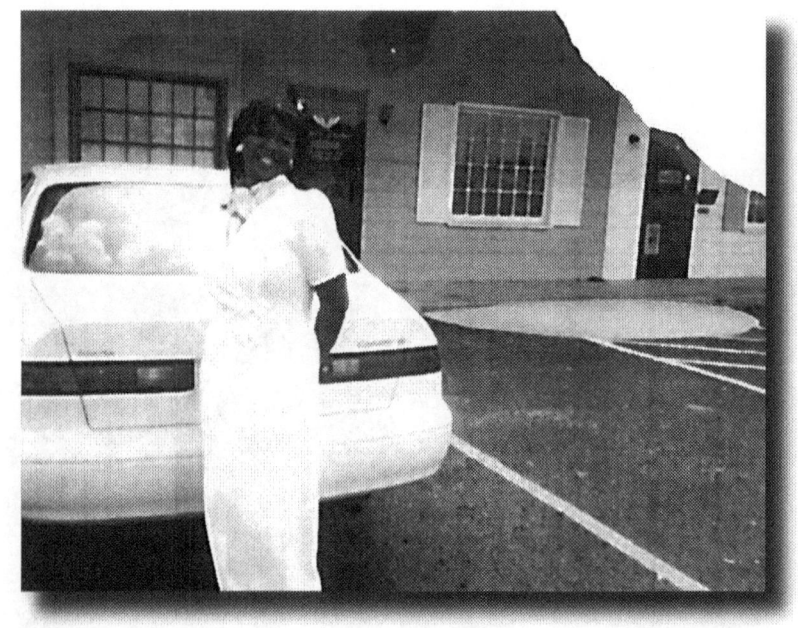

Addie L. Robinson
At
Size 12

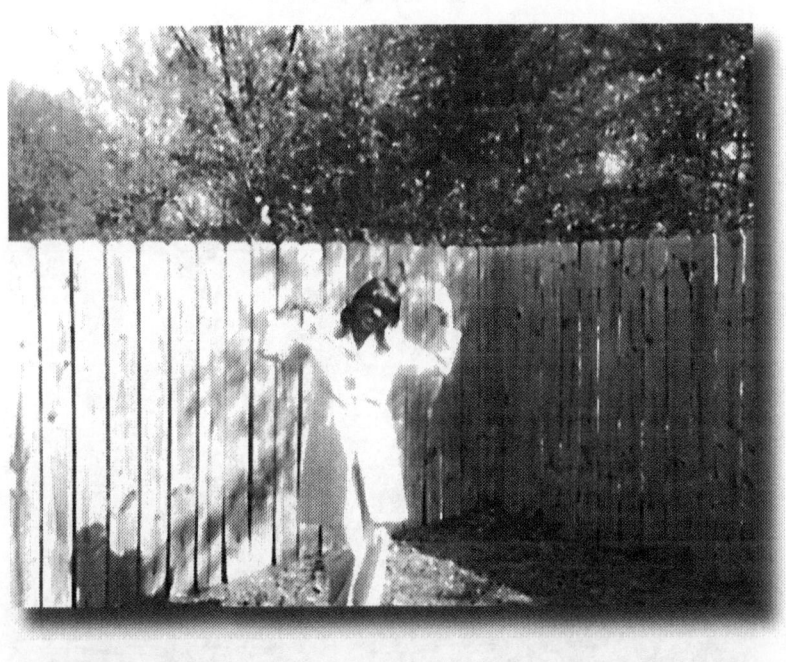

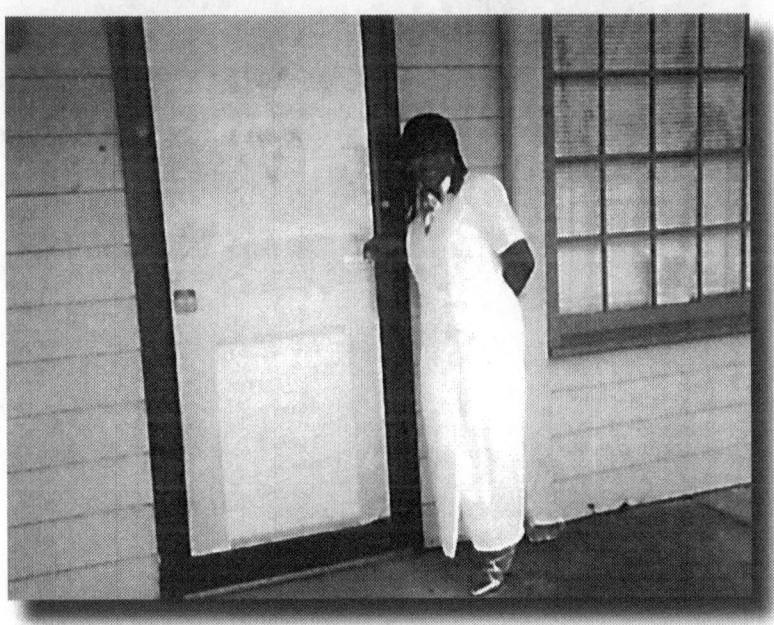

After

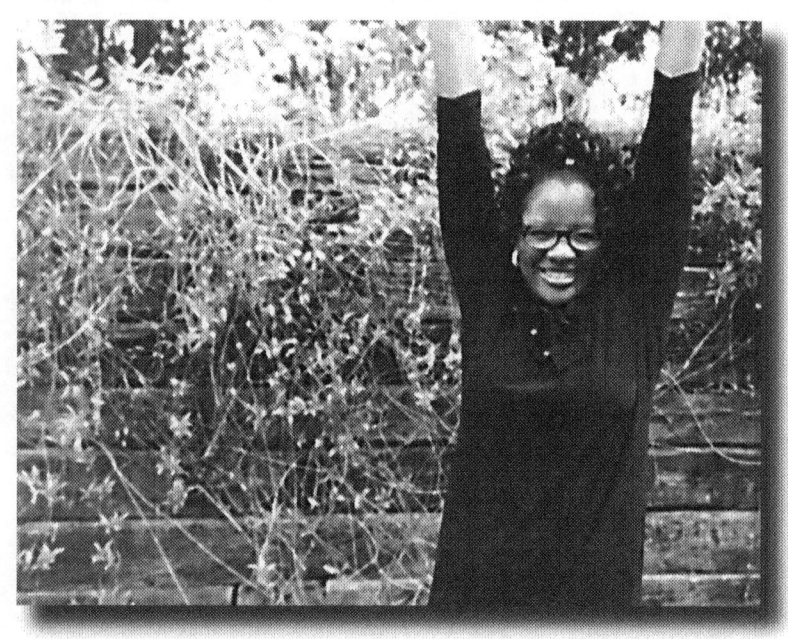

Addie L. Robinson
At
Size 8-10

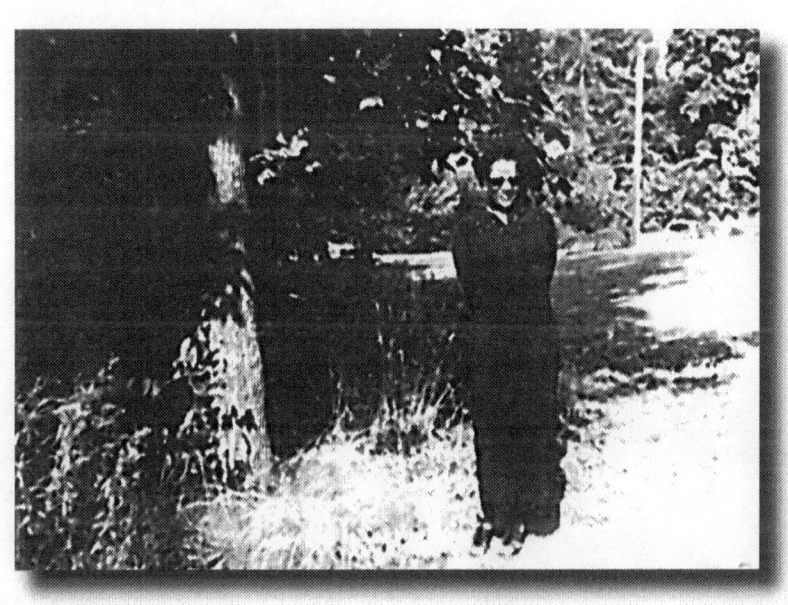

Introduction

In writing this book, I took many things into consideration. One main thing was my motive; what am I writing this book for? The answer I thought of was that there are so many overweight people in this world and all they need is a little push, a little motivation, and a whole lot of determination. This seems to be the thing that the average person trying to lose weight falls short on. So, as I introduce myself, the author, and a weight watcher myself to you, the reader, I would like you to know that I was in the same weight loss battle as some of you are, and through the fight, I became wiser and have realized that there is more to me than meets the eye. I discovered that I'm stronger than I look and I can do more than I ever thought I could. Just when I thought everything was over and I was destined to weigh 232 pounds, and wearing a size 22 forever, I finally began to see the light at the end of the tunnel. Shedding pounds and inches I never thought I could, after trying for years and years to lose the weight. This evidently was my time to drop the weight. I so desperately wanted to lose and as you either continue or begin, according to your purpose of reading this book, to lose your weight. I strongly encourage you to stay strong, know, believe and trust that you can defeat everything that will come your way. Hopefully this is your time to lose your weight as I said before, it took me years to even be productive as far as losing weight. I gave up, and I gave up, but that wasn't the right thing to do now that I look back but we should all learn from our mistakes. So, as you read on, I hope you will get at least one thing that will help you to continue your race to win your prize, which is your weight loss. Even if you have not begun, maybe you can read something in this book to at least get your motor started and when you have finished, I desire nothing but the best for you and yours, and hopefully you will keep on and fulfill your purpose of losing weight. Sit back, relax and enjoy, as you read a book that can bring insight, encouragement and inspire you to get your weight where you want it to be and keep it there.

DEDICATION

As I thought about who to dedicate this book to, it wasn't long before I made my decision. I began to remember when I was injured and suffering with seemingly no one to really support me like I needed. It was a horrible time for me which I felt would never end but it did and I have come so far since then and have accomplished things that I thought could never be done. I guess you can say you shouldn't always go by what you think but by what you know. One thing I do know is that physical injuries, sickness, and permanent impairments aren't anything to laugh about and this is why I chose to dedicate this book to people who are, and have been injured in the past, whether it was in an accident by car, plane, train, bus on your job, or what they call a freak accident, I dedicate this book to you. You are indeed special, because I realize that some accidents may have left some of you, the readers, in many bad situations and with may other sorrows which may or may not have been your fault. In my choosing to dedicate this book to you, I sincerely hope that you take my dedicating this book to you as a vote of confidence. You have someone who is supporting your weight loss efforts and has carefully chosen every topic, every paragraph, every sentence, every word that it might edify and enhance everything you do concerning your weight loss. So, I salute you and admonish you to keep up the good work and move on to possess all the things in life that are rightfully yours.

Contents

Chapter 1

The Beginning Stages of the Transformation Process

Things all began when I least expected it, a time when I had no thoughts of losing weight, or anything to that nature. I was going about my usual day of doing what I wanted, as well as eating what I wanted. Eating usually included restaurants, some more of that, a lots more of this, dinner at all times of the night, fast food anytime I wanted it. Or either I would throw something on the stove, or in the microwave, and eat until I didn't want any more.

But if I could just reflect back on the time before I became pregnant. I wore a size 7/8 clothes at all times. No matter what I ate, when I ate it, a size seven to eight dress or pants would always fit me. This, of course, went on from my teen years until I became pregnant. The perfect size 7/8, I should have modeled at the time, but it never really dawned on me. I was so shapely and able to attract guy's attention at any given time. But those were the good old days.

So now it's time to come to the reality of the fact that it wasn't easy going from a size 22 to a size 10, no indeed, it was hard, grueling work at the beginning, and I know that it has to be just that for so many others who have traveled down this same road of what some folks call getting the fat off. But before we talk about getting the fat off, lets talk about how I, as well as you, the reader, may have gotten the fat on.

I just wrote a little about eating habits. Your eating habits can make you or break you, but of course you know that. Which means, you are going to reflect what you eat at some time or another in your life, whether you eat right everyday, or eat at the right times, consume the proper amount of calories per day, drink everything you should drink

It started by letting myself go, no real restraints on what I ate, fried foods, salty foods, junk foods, etc. But at the time, I wasn't realizing that I was stirring up a Pandora's Box for later on. I didn't realize it was going to be a time of struggling to get the same weight off for 20 years I didn't realize that I was going to have to take the same pounds back off, inch by inch, minute by minute, and day by day. All because I enjoyed eating what I wanted, and when I wanted. This was my past time, going out to dinner.

The days of my size 7/8 were over so I thought nobody was looking anymore, not seriously looking. It seemed like I just got lost in the meals, because when I got dressed and went out to dinner, I was all right as long as I went somewhere. I felt like this was fulfilling an empty void in my life. It may not have been a date but I was going out, size 22 and all. Still never realizing that the same foods I was gobbling down at these nice little restaurants, I was going to have to get back off. I was going to have to go cold turkey, stone cold turkey; no fried chicken, no salty foods, no fatback in my greens, no two and three helpings, but stone cold turkey.

Please don't misinterpret me; there is nothing wrong with going out to restaurants, if you know how to eat properly. But I didn't, I thought this was a time to eat what I want, I'm paying for it. And, I paid dearly. But as I mentioned at the beginning of this book, this was a day I least expected to even try to lose weight. I had tried for years, I prayed, believed God was going to help me, but who would have thought it would have taken all of these years.

The first thing that happened was that I took a good hard look in the mirror at myself. I had taken a hard look before, but it was something about this time. The same face was there, the same 232 pounds was there, but I looked and saw that I could do it if I

of weight. My mind automatically went back to when I heard doctors, as well as other people, tell me how salt sometimes put extra weight on you. But this wasn't the first thing I wanted to do. I thought I couldn't cook any food without salt, perish the thought. I must have been crazy to think I could do this; it was going to take too much. Give up salt, no way. Nevertheless, it had to be done, no matter what. This was one of the first things that needed to be conquered. So, as I took things day by day, my conscious began to nag me every time I ate something with salt in it. But it nagged me, knowing that this was the thing I needed to defeat. I began to reason with myself, and said, self, now you know you have to give up this salt, so you might as well go all the way. From then on, I made a conscious effort not to eat anything else with salt in it. But I began to read certain materials about salt, and I realized that your body needs a certain amount to function properly. So that meant that I just had to watch my salt intake, not eat it as much. I realized that I didn't have to have it on everything I ate, and that I could eat it moderately. Without using half the box to satisfy my taste buds.

It was at that time I began to think more about doctor's reports concerning ailments that can come on you when you over indulge yourself in eating excess amounts of salt. Those reports became important to me. It seemed like thins started coming back to me; things I had heard years ago when I was taught at home about salt intake.

I was no longer out of control, but in control of my salt intake habits and for once feeling like this thing could be done, and smelling the sweet smell of success. But, of course, you know this was just the beginning. My next mountain to climb was fried foods and red meats. OF course, in my mind, I'm automatically thinking, now this is just asking for a little bit too much. I was raised up on fried chicken, fried pork chops, fried hamburgers, and steaks. If it was fried, I ate it. How could I do this, how could I stop this tradition? How could I put the frying pan down, and learn hot to eat baked, grilled or stewed foods instead. This was indeed the challenge of the year. But again, it had to be done. At first I eased up on the chicken since this was my favorite, with hot sauce. It felt like I just couldn't do it. Every time I went to eat in a restaurant, or at home, I still had to have me some fried chicken. But this didn't go on much longer, before I had another talk with myself. I thought I had come so far, I had already conquered one of the most enslaving problems, which was the salt intake so I said, Addie, you can do this thing. Time went past and the more I tried to eat friend foods, the more my taste buds dissolved for it. It almost seemed like when I went around fried foods, I went the other way. It wasn't easy but I knew that I wasn't going to be able to resist the temptation if I stayed around it. So again I made up my mind one day that I was going to lose the weight, and that I had come too far, and I wasn't going to allow a bowl of deeply golden browned cooked to perfection chicken stop me. I had to walk away every time. It wasn't easy but I did it. It took all the will power I had, but I did it. So after this, I began to see the weight falling off. Inches fell of, pounds fell off, and I don't think I had been that happy for a while. This was the moment I had been waiting for, a size 20. Then I went down to a size 18. This was fantastic, it was hard, but it was fantastic. I couldn't believe my eyes. I got rid of clothes, anything resembling a size 22. I was making it. The battle was really on.

But that didn't stop me. I began to look at the packages of everything I ate. I wanted to know how much of everything was in it, as if I had been to school for a nutritionist or something. But if the numbers looked too high, I put it back on the shelf. If the numbers looked like it was something nutritional for my body, then I bought it. I can't say that I knew everything, but again, I went back to what I had already heard the doctors say for years and heard through the grapevine. Take care of your bodies, watch what you eat. At this point my mind had changed because if I could lay off the salt and fried foods, I could do anything. This is not to say that I did it on my own. I know that God guided me through the whole ordeal and that I was going to be the one going to come out with the prize. The prize of my body being healthy, feeling young again, able to do things I wasn't able to do physically when I was weighing 232 pounds.

My ship must have finally come in because the next thing I took on was the amount of food I ate per day. This wasn't easy for me because, remember, I'm the one that ate all times of the night, even though I had a lot of heartburn and even chest pain at times. But I would drink warm water and baking soda and think all of problems were going away. This also was something that had to be done, and baking soda and warm water couldn't help me then. So as I began to tackle this problem, it seemed the more I didn't eat at night, the more I wanted to eat at night, mostly 10:00 pm, even later sometimes, after I knew the usual time for eating your last meal. But, once again, I was determined that I had come too far. I had started looking better, talking better, and walking better, and that's all I needed to see. So I kept on encouraging myself and when the evening came and time for me to eat my last meal of the day, I started making sure it was something I wanted, and that I was going to be satisfied. But in between meals, I sometimes ate fruit; bananas, apples, oranges, grapes or Kiwis, as well as drank juice, making sure I read the back of the labels again, being able to see how much nutrition I was putting into my body each day.

In addition to all this, I already had begun to exercise, walk and even found a place to work out. All of this did me a world of good. Strangely enough, it all became fun to me. I began to set times when I was going to walk, when I was going to work out and when I was going to exercise. Then to take things even further, I learned how to eat healthy foods. I read books and magazines. I didn't eat all the things I used to. When I went in restaurants, I ordered grilled chicken instead of fried chicken. Sometimes I might have slipped up and ate a piece of fried chicken here and there. But it was no more fried pork chops, hamburger, steak or other fried foods that were going to cause me to go out of control. No, indeed.

I acquired a taste for mainly eating grilled, stewed, or baked meats. Then I had a taste for salads. I started making up my own salads, as long as it looked like it was going to be good for me, I tried it. Salads were never on my list of things to eat, but it quickly became one of my favorites. I was not making a discovery that there was a whole other world of foods that I could enjoy. I didn't have to eat fried chicken 3-4 times a week. I could bake it, grill it or stew it. Of course, without all of the salt. This was just amazing to me. After 20 years of struggling with the same weight problem, I was finally seeing the light at the end of the tunnel. There was hope after all.

By this time I had come down to a size 16. Can you believe it? Me, a size 16. Nobody was going to ever believe this, but it was true. I knew what fully in control meant. I had come a long way because before I thought I knew what in control meant but now I was fully in control. Because in my eating habits, I had developed a new level of self-control, I looked better, I felt better, yes indeed, this is it. No more teasing, no more uneasiness around other people because of my weight. I had slayed the dragons in my life that kept me eating, and eating. And I did it without medications, without being stressed out, without feeling bound up by diets. For once I took control and won the battle. It wasn't the prettiest victory, but it was mine. I win, I get my life back, I get another chance, a chance to be healthy, to encourage someone else, and say if I can drop 83 pounds and counting, then so can you.

The expression of my saying I'm glad the weight is off does not even touch the surface of what losing this weight has done for me. My whole life has changed because of it. If I can do it, so can you. Don't give up now; there is still hope for you yet. If you followed me in this chapter, what did I say I did? I first of all made up my mind that this could be done. Then, I settled it in my heart, and then I went to work. I stopped all the unnecessary salt. Then I worked on the fried foods, which was the most difficult task of all, but if I can do it so can you. Then I also discussed eating at the right times; conquering that dragon and then earlier I wrote to you concerning resting. I didn't really tell you how grueling it was for me to exercise. I was lazy. My body was tired all of the time from carrying all of the weight. It was so difficult at the beginning, just getting my motor started. I would exercise one day and didn't do anything for days, but at that time, my ship had come in. Either I was going to get on board and ride, or I was going to let it go past. So, as I got the energy, and the mind to go on with this weight loss thing, I kept riding the wave. It didn't happen over night. I worked at it and I worked at it, and I was rewarded for my diligence. I'm a size 10 and ready to go back to a 7/8 now, and still enjoying the fruits of my labor.

I also realize that if I had not developed character along with losing the weight, I would be right back on the sidelines looking, waiting for another opportunity to board a ship that might not ever come again. When I say character, I mean self-control, appreciation for who I really am. I am now realizing that if I could get all of this weight off after 18 years, then I can go on to defeat the rest of the things in my life that I thought could never be done. This, I think, was one of the biggest and toughest challenges for me in my life. Giving up the foods I loved so much was devastating. But in the midst of it all, I have learned that what I see in front of me does not compare to what is behind the wall; that is hidden from me. In this case, it was the relief of back, leg and neck pain almost every day. I also had an injury to my right ankle. But when I began to lose the weight, the pain in my back subsided, my legs didn't hurt and feel like jelly when I walked anymore or when I went up and down the stairs. I haven't been waking up in the middle of the night with neck pain. My right ankle gives me less problems, and I have begun to wear heels again in moderation, of course. So we see that not only did I find out some things about myself but also my body was getting more out of it than just weight loss. These were things I did not do when the doctors explained them to me years ago or when I read magazines and saw health programs on television. I was just too lazy and greedy. I wanted what I wanted when I wanted it. I was out of control. I wouldn't hear of getting off the salt, or make a conscious effort of getting the weight off, but it cost me. For years of my life I was overweight, and if I would have just done this then, I probably could have accomplished more with my life. Because my injuries limited me, I wont' say that I never have pain, but I will say that as I am cautious, still watching what I eat, and keeping my body in shape, that my pain has lessened so much that I sometimes don't even remember that I had injured myself in the past. This is not to say that things would work this way for you. You may have never had any injuries and had your physician tell you to do these things, but you still want to lose weight. Your self-esteem may be low; people teased you until you were in tears, called you names, and made you feel bad about yourself. So you started viewing yourself negatively because of the weight and what people said. But I say the same thing I have been saying all along, if I can do it, you can do it too. Whatever reason you want to lose weight is your own reason, but if you're like me, you want to but just think you can't. Maybe you fell off the wagon so many times that you don't even want to ride anymore. So what do I say to that? I say it's strictly your decision to stay in your state, or dig down deep inside yourself, and make the effort to lose the weight. Maybe you just might come up with more than you bargained for, like I did, with the lessening of pain in the back, legs, neck, and ankle. This was something I could have done all along, but couldn't see past the walls of laziness, greediness, no self-control, overlooking the needs of my body, rather than making sure I was healthy. I'm not saying I eat everything right every day, but I'm in charge of what goes in my body and I also realize that what goes into my body, I am totally responsible for later. Because nobody twisted my arm and made me eat that way. I was unconsciously enjoying myself. Unconscious because when I look back, I wasn't realizing what I was doing. I was just doing what I thought was natural. Fried chicken all of the time, soda all day long, eating when I wanted. This was the norm, but in reality, it really wasn't the norm. Because I was hurting myself in more ways than one. But all along I still was praying that God would keep me through this and He did. Not only did He keep me through it, but I received a little mercy too because there were times when I wanted to say, am I sure I'm doing the right thing here or is this another pipe dream. Then a few people said to me, that's enough weight off now, you're losing too much. But that's when it seemed like He reminded me that, if you want to reach your goals, then you have to keep on moving and so I did. And the result of that is a size 10 and counting, a better attitude, a healthier body, back, leg neck and ankle pain tremendously subsiding if you want to see mercy in action then this was it and what I deem to be a bonified miracle. I was supposedly doomed to being a size 22 and counting, not liking the way I looked but seemingly couldn't do anything about it. But evidently that wasn't true, and even though people felt like I had done enough, but this was my battle to fight. And so, I say the same to you who think you can't win the battle. The battle can be won, and you can be the one who wins it, just by making up your mind, and putting your best foot forward. This includes digging down inside yourself, and finding those things that are going to propel you to a point of saying I can make it if I try.

Strengthening your will power always helps. Resisting things that are not going to help your cause, arming yourself with plenty of information about your body, how to care for it, what it needs to survive, etc. But most of all, take a good hard look in the mirror and decide why you are wanting to lose weight, what do you have to do to get the job done, and don't forget to find your own faults, where you are lacking in areas such as self control, over eating, or laziness. You do this because this is going to help you find your way through the maze of the weight loss battle. You'll know where your weak points are, and your strong points are, and where you should focus your attention the most. You are going to have to be confronted as well as the weight dragon, if you want to accomplish your goal. You're going to have to fight for it. For some it may be easier than others but the result will be the same. If you don't like the size you are, only you can change it. I didn't win my battle until I thoroughly, one hundred and ten percent, made up my mind to conquer this thing called fat. It took sweat and sometimes tears, but if I can do it so can you. And I strongly suggest that you don't do it for someone else. I strongly suggest that you do it for yourself. So that you will feel good about yourself, you will be healthy; you can find that life is worth living and that you can now tap into your inner strength, which is inside all of us. If we learn how to master this thing called will power, we can and will avoid a lot of traps and pitfalls set before us. So now I say to you, reader, that the ball is in your court. Either you are going to play, or you're going to let it get away, the weight problem, that is. But if you think that you have let it get away too long, then maybe this could be your day. Maybe this could be your turn around point. I'm certainly hoping that reading this chapter, and this entire book, is one of the best things that has ever happened to you. That you have looked at yourself and made a conscious positive decision to lose the weight that has been plaguing your life. But if this one chapter has not been enough to convince you, then you don't want to miss these next chapters. A lot of thought and time has went into them, and they are specifically designed to allow you, the reader, to shape the next level of my journey to losing every inch and pound of your unwanted weight. So sit back, grab a healthy snack and enjoy.

CHAPTER 2

Meeting the Challenge

When I first noticed that my weight was getting out of control, it was the year 1980. I was pregnant and told that this was the normal thing, that pregnant women automatically gained weight. So, if I could say anything, I guess I just let everything go past my head at that very moment as I ate more and more. I had already rehearsed it in my mind that I'm pregnant; the baby is going to put a little extra weight on me. It'll come off. I realize I'm going to eat extra everything, so I'll just wait until I have the baby and then I'll work on the weight situation. As you know, months went on and as my stomach got bigger, so did I. I didn't really focus that much on my weight at the time, but I knew that it was becoming a problem fast. Still, in the back of my mind was, I'll wait until I have the baby and then I'll deal with the weight situation. But boy how wrong could I be. I strongly believe that this was my turning point for my weight gain problem. As I basically said in the previous chapter, I was out of control. This is where everything could have possibly begun. I thought it was the norm and I just lit it ride, and probably did things in excess. I should have eaten less, but then I was concerned about my unborn child. Are they getting all the nourishment that they should if I eat less?

These were some of the questions that nagged at me at the beginning, but again, I didn't pay it a whole lot of attention. I had already determined when I was going to handle the situation; it was set and planned in my mind. Now I realize that all I had to do was discuss it further with my doctor and I probably could have gotten more direction and understanding about what, and how much to eat. But at that time, I was kind of young and didn't have a lot of clear direction of my own life, let alone talking about having a child. The only thing I knew was that I wanted my child to be healthy.

Time went past and my baby was delivered. It was a girl. Needless to say that once I had my daughter, I sought help for my weight gain problem. I went to doctor after doctor just hoping that they would give me a pill to make the fat go away. They all gave me the same advice. Watch what you eat, exercise and get your proper rest. But that wasn't the story I wanted to hear. My ideal story was; take this with plenty of water, call me in the morning and all of the weight will be gone.

So then, here comes discouragement ready to take over, ready to make me give up. This went on for years, waiting for someone to give me an easy way out and there was none. While I went on the chase for the right pill, the right doctor, the so-called right solution, it seemed like I was gaining more weight by the minute. It wasn't fair. When I was carrying the baby, I had it all planned out. I was going to get it all off, it wasn't going to even be a problem. I was going to change back into all of my previous eating habits and I was going to exercise. What happened to me? Was I tricked into thinking that I had time, that the weight was just a temporary set back, that I didn't need to do anything but ride on easy street? I guess the answer to all of this is yes. I was tricked into thinking I was going to get my body and my eating habits back.

How was I going to deal with this? I was getting no answers from the doctors now; not anything I really wanted to hear. So I thought I couldn't find a secret potion. Where was I going to begin now? Discouragement was setting in and seemingly I didn't have a chance at losing all of this unwanted weight. As I said, years were going by and I was getting worse and worse, bigger and bigger.

This wasn't exactly what I had in mind. I wanted my body back. I never really realized that the answer was inside of me; the ability to bring what I wanted to pass was inside of me. So I began to feel like this was just never going to happen. I was supposed to be this size, the weight wasn't coming off, and I give up. There was no answer to this problem, so as time went on, I began to look older than I was. I began to feel older than I was. I was tired all of the time, sweating, hot and irritated when I walked one block. My legs hurt so bad until sometimes I wouldn't even try to go anywhere because I knew they were going to bother me. I knew I wasn't going to walk very far. Hopes of me losing the weight were beginning to look slim and none, so I thought.

When I went back to the doctor, it was still the same answer. You have to lose the weight. But it seemed like the more they said that, the more I rebelled, the more I wanted what I wanted, when I wanted it. So, I guess you can see that at this point I was bringing things on myself. Not doing what I was advised, considering my own wants and desires first rather than the needs of my body. My body, at this time, needed major attention but I wanted someone else to do it. I wanted a quick fix and that just wasn't going to happen.

In addition to all of my weight woes, I still had a child to contend with. I still had to give her what she needed. Needless to say, emotionally, I had put myself in a web. I knew I had to keep a clear head in order to care for my child. But at the same time, this weight thing was taking a toll on me. I was tired of being tired physically, as well as mentally. I was having an inner battle you would not have believed. My self-esteem became damaged as I tried to lose the weight.

This wasn't the way I want to look; this wasn't the weight I wanted to be. I was unhappy with myself, with my appearance and yet feeling trapped by foods. This was no way for anyone to live. Unhappy and really not exemplifying all of the necessary qualities to make sure a child has a healthy life. I strongly believe in order for a child to be well rounded and healthy, the parent must give 110% of themselves. But I was falling short and I knew I had to do something about myself. What could I do? It seemed to be over. The weight was remaining, all of my will power was gone, and my mind wasn't even computing trying to lose the weight anymore. So as I said before, I gave up. I was not realizing that what I really wanted was on the other side of the wall of discouragement, hopelessness, and tiredness, physically as well as mentally.

As years went by I just fell in the overweight pit like so many others and as foods dominated my life, my child grew and so did I. Pound after pound. But the sad part was, it was never that I stopped caring about the weight loss problem, or myself but I felt bound by this thing called lack of self-control.

This is where I missed the mark. My mind told me I couldn't go any further, I couldn't accomplish what I was trying to do, I might as well give up. You look okay like this, not as good as before, but you'll live. But even though these thoughts settled in my mind, it was almost as if somewhere deep inside of me, I still wanted to get my life back. It just didn't seem right that I couldn't lose the weight. It seemed so simple, all I had to do was slack up on the eating, get my diet in order, right? But it never worked out quite that way after I had my child.

As time went on, in some way I became accustomed to getting bigger and bigger. I would shop for clothes with almost no kind of a feeling about it after a while. I was moving up the ladder in sizes, 10,

12, 14, 16, 18, 20 and 22. This was ridiculous but still I had no power to fight back. It wasn't that I wasn't putting forth any effort but I was out of control.

I was still not taking medical advice, even after having injuries to my neck and back. I went through therapy, but that didn't help the weight problem. That seemed to be in a category all of its own. Either I was going to do it or I wasn't, because I was going nowhere fast.

So there I was; hurting all of the time, tired in my body and carrying a major problem that wouldn't go away. I remember joining a church after a while, not for weight loss purposes but because this was what I wanted. I didn't even ask God right away about the weight. I just went faithfully and enjoyed the services. But somewhere in between going to church and struggling with the weight loss, I heard somebody say, if you just ask God to help you, He will. So I started to pray. I began asking God to help me with the weight loss problem. I told Him I couldn't do it. I didn't know where to begin anymore, that I didn't have any more will power, that this thing was just impossible.

I'd like to say that He came right in and turned it all around but it didn't happen that way. I kept crying out to Him, asking Him to help me with the weight loss. I was still out of control, still eating what I wanted and doing what I wanted to do. This was confusing because why wasn't He just knocking the weight off? I mean He's God, right? It was still years and years of going past that I kept asking God. Finally I stopped asking and changed the tide. I began to thank Him for helping me, even though I didn't see the weight loss yet. And as I kept on thanking Him, I began getting a peace about things but things still didn't go like I wanted them to. The weight was still there and I had to bear it, as much as I wanted to go back to my original size before I had become pregnant.

I kept on living and waiting for something to happen with much anticipation, but this opened the door for my patience level to go down to zero. And through it all, a peace about things was still there. After I stopped asking God to fix the situation, it seemed like it was time to move on to other issues in my life. Still, there was no sign of anything happening. I was still eating like there was no tomorrow and was seemingly out of the race to meet a decent man, not even mentioning the fact that almost everybody I socialized with was slimmer than myself. I guess this didn't help either. They often encouraged me about the weight but it never seemed to be enough. Then there were those that teased and jokingly called me names. I guess they weren't realizing that their words were hurting more than helping to get the weight off, heavily damaging my self-esteem. And at that particular time I didn't know any better, I allowed this to happen to me. When people spoke negative, hurtful things to me, I held in my true feelings and laughed along with the joke, knowing that I wanted to burst into tears. But I held that until I was alone and kept crying out to God. Maybe I should forget about this God thing too. Maybe He wasn't going to help me after all. Of course these were the thoughts that were going through my mind at the time. But I know that wasn't true, because of all the things I had learned about Him, and how He had proved Himself in so many other situations. God was not going to let me down. But after years of waiting and waiting, I should have felt that way, and at some point and time during the waiting period, I did give up on God. I was thinking I might as well forget Him, He's not even going to help me. But I'd usually end up forgetting about feeling like that and once again forgot about the weight loss problem.

Now, to bring you up to the year 1998, in the month of August, still desiring to lose the weight, but feeling trapped inside. Even with the encouragement, things still weren't working. Until one day I looked in the mirror and saw who I didn't want to be anymore. Day after day I would see something else I wanted changed. I knew I could look better. I knew I had it in me to carry myself better, to look my very best. But sometimes when I looked, it still seemed like it couldn't be done. It was too much hard work because I supposedly had went down too far. I had too many pounds to lose. The money just wasn't there for diet pills, spas and extra foods that would take off the fat. I was too tired all of the time to walk and exercise. The pain in my back and neck was so bad at times that I couldn't lift things, bend over, or walk very far.

These were the many excuses I used, not realizing that if I didn't do it then, when was a good time? Was I waiting for the perfect time? Was I waiting for more money? Was I waiting until my body was better? If I was waiting for any of these things, I was about to miss out. The time was then, and God was finally showing up. But how was I going to pull this off? Where was I going to get the money, how long was my back, neck, legs and ankle going to hold up when I begin to exercise and walk? These were all of the questions in my mind, but now that I think about it, none of the questions were important. They didn't have anything to do with anything. Either I was going to get what I had been waiting for or I wasn't. So I stopped focusing on how I was going to get the money or how my body was going to hold up, and began to take things day by day.

This was how I started meeting the challenge, taking things day by day, not cluttering my mind with tomorrow, the week, or even the next month. My focus became; what can I do to lose a few more pounds today. How can I change myself all the way around? It was then that I decided to go all of the way. I might as well lose weight, look better, and feel better. This was the challenge of a lifetime for me. Here I am 232 pounds, no will power, so it seemed, and no real finances to get the job done.

Here I am, talking about changing my entire world. So, after this time of looking in the mirror and seeing someone that I didn't want to be anymore, it was finally time to change, after 18 years of struggling with the same thing, it was definitely time to push myself until the job was completed. Completed, meaning until I'm satisfied, not really even considering anyone else but God and myself. I needed to come to the point of liking and loving myself. It was going to be a difficult task for me, but I somehow knew it could be done. Everything finally was going to be all right. So I took on the challenge.

It was rocky at the beginning. I had to adjust my thinking from; I can't do this, to, I will do this. I had to tell myself over and over and over again that this was it, and I had to do this. It seemed like now was a good time to dig into a part of me that I had forgotten existed, a part of my character that was buried when discouragement came, when the giving up came, when everything went down hill. I was always a determined person, someone that was determined to get what they wanted. In some kind of way, determination rose up in me, the more things tried to get away from me, the more determined I became. Things like eating healthy, exercising, watching my weight. These were the very same things that I neglected to do when advised by my physician in the beginning.

I could have saved myself 18 years of heartache, disappointment and discouragement. How wrong could I have been? Eating healthy, working out, watching my diet wasn't so bad after all. In fact, I began to make it fun. I created new dishes and took walks where there was scenery. I met new people at the gym and it became an adventure because this was a whole new world for me.

This was the same person that thought it couldn't be done. The one that gave up and thought that God must have forgotten about her. Now, watching her mind change, her attitude change, her body change, but most of all her life changing. Talking about meeting the challenge - this was it.

Taking things day by day was one of the keys. Another key was to fight for what I wanted because even though you, as the reader, and even myself, want things to be rosy and peaches and cream. It just doesn't happen that way. We have to work for what we want, resist the temptations and conquer those things that are going to be a hindrance to us. That's the only way we are going to achieve our goals. I didn't lose 83 pounds, and counting, easy. I had to be strong, willing to exercise my mind, my will power and defeat and conquer everything that came my way.

Like I said, it wasn't easy, I was down in a slump with this weight loss thing. At one time, as far as I was concerned, it was over. But I know now that the prayer made all the difference. For the simple reason I couldn't bring myself back to life. I needed a resurrection. Everything in me was buried. I thought I was doomed to a size 22, but even thought things took years, I came out with the victory over the weight and I'm going to keep the victory over the weight.

I still have goals to meet and I'm going to meet every last one of them. This weight loss ordeal has taught me a valuable lesson and I'm going to go throughout the rest of my life doing what is best for me. I realize I'm going to make mistakes, but I accept the challenge and whatever I want is mine.

So as you continue to conquer those dragons in your life, remember you might have to fight, scratch and claw, but hang in there until you reach your ultimate goal, I say ultimate because you might want to stop in the middle of your challenge. Because we sometimes thinking we can't get past the dragon, we can't get past the wall, but if we keep on moving in spite of the dragon, then we get to win the prize. In this case, the prize was my weight loss, my self-esteem, my youth, and my health. I had to meet the challenge. Even though I might have wanted them to, no one else was going to meet my challenge. I had to face this dragon on my own, along with the help of my Lord and Savior Jesus Christ. We did it without drugs, without a mountain of money, and without the advantages that other people might have had. So, if you say that it can't be done, you can't lose the weight, or once you lost it, you gain it right back. Then you might need to examine yourself. You gain it right back only because you allow yourself to. You may have won the prize but sometimes the war goes on. You still might have to resist certain foods, certain people you know that will negatively affect what you are doing, but if you have successfully conquered those dragons then you are the one in control. What you say stands, and whatever you do and allow yourself to fall prey to stands also. You still have a choice in the matter, whether you are going to stay in charge or let yourself go again is up to you. The ball is in your court. A reality check should show you that all you have to do is remember where you came from and that should be enough to keep you motivated. Turning back should not even be an option for you. You can build yourself up to a point where you won't turn around no matter what. And, if you do decide to turn around, you have another way to start all over again. Weight loss is not a game. It's something that could mean so much more than just losing weight. Everything about you may be hanging in the balance. Your very life could be at stake, and you don't know which way to turn but if you take a good hard look at yourself, you just might see your way out. Then you might gather enough courage to make your steps day by day. You are able to slay your dragons and bring them under your subjection, under your control. You can start exercising your will power. This forgotten inner powerful force was my greatest asset. It was something I very seldom used, very seldom heard anyone talk about, but it was there inside of me, waiting to be activated, waiting to help me meet the challenge. I didn't even realize it was so important until I tried to lose the weight, and couldn't figure out what was wrong. I couldn't figure out why I was out of control, why I went in the restaurants and ate until my heart was content, without any restraints. I needed something. It wasn't a pill, it wasn't a lot of fad dieting, and it wasn't starving myself until I was sick, but it was a void that needed to be filled. Make no mistake about it. If this is the way you choose to lose your weight, then that's not my decision to make, but it's yours. But I chose another way, and that way was will power and self-control. After I caught on to the revelation that it was all about will power and self-control, I grabbed a hold of it and haven't let it go since then. It's been keeping me at my size 10 and slowly meeting my goal of a size 7/8.

The void had finally been filled, after 18 years of struggling, shame, tiredness, disappointment and discouragement. I'm not saying that this was all it took because for me, it took this and some more. But these were the major tools being used to help me over my mountain of weight. Like I said, it was a time I felt trapped, and just gave up but when I learned to resist the food I was so hooked on that was luring me, or when I went into my favorite restaurant, not to order something fried, but order something grilled or baked. It was then that I had begun to use these two powerful forces already invested in me from the beginning. I know that we all have these inner forces in us to help us through life, called self-control, and will power to not do what we don't want to do. If the person that wants to lose weight wouldn't eat because they don't want to eat, then they can meet their goals and lose all the weight that they need to, whether it be for health reasons or not. If you think about it, it's either you're going to do something or you're not. Let's face it, it's not the easiest thing to just say no, but it can be done.

CHAPTER 3

There Is Hope for You After All

When we think about the word hope, we may think of something happening in spite of the odds against it happening. For example, when the doctor might have said that a loved one may not make it, but there's always someone in the family that says, they're strong, they can do it, they'll come out of it. But still, the person may end up passing on anyway. But in spite of that one person still hoped until the very end. So hope is not something that is taken lightly, but hope can keep you thriving when others have given up and thrown in the towel. Like so many of us, and like myself at one time, we have given up hope in shedding those pounds we so desperately need to get off. We have hung up our sneakers and called it quits. Our hope has diminished to absolutely nothing. That's why we eat and eat and eat. We have traded our hope in for the foods we love, for our lazy ways, for the unwillingness to take care of our bodies. Hope is another powerful force that can get us what we want in this weight loss fight, because if hopelessness can knock us out, it will. Hopelessness takes all of our vision, all of our goals and all of our insight. If we have no hope, we can't see the forest for the trees. We can't see that we can drop those 50, 60, 70, 80, or 90 pounds we need to drop. But we say that I tried and I tried and this weight loss thing is just not going to happen. I've spent X amount of dollars and worked out until I can't work out anymore. So they fall off the wagon, and gain even more weight, but this time the hopelessness, the negative attitude and the unwillingness to go on becomes a part of them and they never go any further. They never accomplish what they set out to do. Therefore, they have wasted all of those days and nights at the gym, their money or whatever else they were doing to lose the weight. But with that same time and effort people use to be hopeless and make excuses, they could be working toward their goals, their health, and making their lives better. Somewhere along the line their minds were changed. I presume it was when things looked too hard, or when they had to sweat a little too much. Whatever the situation, they now have to find a way to get back up on their horse and ride. Just because you get knocked down doesn't mean life is over or that your weight loss goals can't be met. They can be met if you learn the secrets of making sure that we keep hoping and working on our goals at the same time then all we want to do can and will be done. If you take me for instance, I gave u hope on several occasions. Once when I felt overwhelmed and outdone by my weight loss situation, I couldn't foresee anything but what I was seeing, it seemed like it was no use going on, because after all, I had tried to do this very same thing for so long that it was becoming ridiculous.

I remember when I first started trying to lose the weight. It seemed easy at first. I would have my baby and then I would lose the weight. This was my master plan, as I said in the previous chapters. It was going to be as simple as one, two, three. Slow down on the eating, slack up on the salt and the sugar, walk a couple blocks and everything was going to be okay. So I slacked up on the eating, the salt, the sugar, and walked a little. But before I knew it, I was doing everything I said I wasn't going to do. I was still doing what I wanted, which definitely didn't help. So of course, what little weight I lost came back and I just knew that this was it. Time to pack it in and give it up. I remember being upset with myself that I couldn't do what I had set out to do. This was not within my character. When I said I was going to do something I usually did it. But there was something about this weight loss thing I couldn't seem to conquer. Even though I was ready, willing, and so I thought able, it just never seemed to happen my way. One week I was, so called, slacked up and the next week I was out of control. This went on for years until I finally just gave up hope of this thing ever happening all together. I threw in the towel; I got sick of myself and gave up. So there I was, big as ever, tired, sweating, body hurting, feeling bad about myself giving up hope. This, I guess, should have been the time to dig my claws in and hang in there. But I made my choice, and that was to give up and allowed myself to stay in the same state.

This wasn't exactly what I wanted to do but as I said before, things seemed so overwhelming and I couldn't see the forest for the trees. But now I see things in a total different light, giving up definitely wasn't the answer then, and never has been the answer to any problem in our lives.

We as human beings tend to do the wrong thing sometimes and fall to the wayside just as some of us might have done with out weight loss woes. I say woes because losing weight is a major problem, sorrow and adventure at times. Either we don't have the patience, or we don't have the money, or we are out of control, or we just don't know where to begin, so we begin nowhere. I would like to say it was easy for me and that once I received the revelation that it was time to deal with my weight that I was more than willing, but that's not true. I had given up, tired of myself, and had become so comfortable with not getting the weight off that it had literally become a part of who I was whether I liked it or not. Even though years and years were going past, and it was stealing who I was. My youth felt drained, I was tired all of the time and as I previously mentioned I had several injuries to myself and wasn't looking my best. I didn't realize it then but life was moving on without me. I didn't really want to be this way, but because my will power was not being used and I was out of control but most of all, I was without understanding of who I really was, and what I really could do if I would must take another route and make the necessary adjustments and sacrifices. So, therefore, as my hope slowly diminished, I lost so much more than just gained extra pounds. I lost a part of myself that only God and myself could really put back together. I realize that I could not have done it without Him but I also realized that He would not have done it without me. So as I end this chapter, please remember that hope is a powerful, powerful key in your failing or succeeding. If you lose it then you have already lost the weight loss game, but if you savor it, your chances increase more and more each day to conquer this weight loss thing. So we see that hope is valuable, not only for losing weight, but for life in general. And if we get knocked off of our weight loss horse but still have a little hope left, then we can get back up and ride again. But if we fall with no hope at all, then there is no guarantee that we are going to get back up. Hope is on the inside of you and if you could just tap into it, this could be a good starting point for you in losing weight. And in the famous words you may have heard before, keep hope alive.

CHAPTER 4

Basking In Your Beauty

I'd like to begin this chapter by discussing you. You as a whole, you as a woman, you as a man, just you as a person in general, someone that has great capabilities. Abel to basically do anything you want if you would apply yourself to it. I don't say this to boost your ego, but I say this to share with you, who thought you couldn't do anything right, that you couldn't even lose the weight if you tried, that we as human beings seem to be capable of accomplishing so much more than we give ourselves credit for. Let's take someone that is overweight and knows their health is in danger if they don't lose the weight at a certain time. This person tends to do what they want, knowing that they have to lose the weight. They eat everything in sight, late hours, knowing that it can still increase the weight problem. But they continue in this reckless manner, possibly hoping that their problems would disappear, but it doesn't, and things get worse. Their health deteriorates; everything that the doctor said was going to happen began to come true. Could you imagine the inner feelings of this person, regret maybe, or perhaps disgust, depression, sad, now thinking to themselves why didn't I listen when I had the chance. Why did I persist to do what I wanted to do in spite of my warnings? Did I think I was going to escape? Did I think this must have been for someone else? My health will not fail me; I'm going to be all right. The doctors don't know everything; I'm feeling all right so far, nothing's going to happen to me. Could you imagine how badly this person would like to have turned back the hands of time and do things all over again? This would be nice but unfortunately life doesn't go that way. Either you're going to do or you are not. But just think, this person could have made another choice. They could have done everything right at the beginning. They could have taken their physician's advice and lost the weight. But this was their own decision, which brings me to this very important point of saying that when we tap into our inner beauty we have a choice, a chance to use what's naturally given to us or not to use it.

Beauty to me is not just for the looks of a female gender. There is also an inner beauty-natural beauty, a beauty we were born with, and it is in all of us. So I'm not just talking about the outward appearance, I'm talking about the part of us that makes us who we are on the inside. Can you think of yourself using every bit of your self-control, making sure you are controlling what's happening in your life and what's not. Controlling your need to excessively eat. Just think, you can do that if you tried. You may say not me. I can't control anything. My children are out of control, my life is out of control, and my eating habits are out of control. I eat night and day. I've already tried to stop but I just can't. But I say that you can still lose weight, whatever your situation may be because one of the keys to self-control is keeping your hope alive. No one else can do it for you. Like my self, I wanted a quick fix. I thought someone else was going to give me a quick solution to my problem but only to find out that there was no quick fix. I had to suffer it out, pound by pound, inch by inch. I had to keep my own hope alive. I had to lean how to master this thing called self-control. It wasn't easy but I have come a long way and I would never tell it that I always have it all together but most of the time I do compared to all of the things that wanted to take me under. I had to conquer them or they were going to conquer me. Self-control didn't' come easy and I had to work at it, but it came and I tapped into it and have been surviving from it ever since.

My battle with self-control might have been totally different from yours, as the reader, but either way, we can possess this great quality called self-control, especially in our eating habits. One main thing that can be done to tame your appetite to resist things that we do want and realize that it would not help your cause for you to eat certain foods that are going to keep the weight on. I could easily have said resist the things that you don't want, but that's not resisting, that's just walking away from what you don't want anyway. There is no challenge in that, but if you can walk away from the food that's calling you in the midnight hour, and resist these foods, which are high in everything, that you're not supposed to eat, then you have accomplished a great goal and you definitely need to celebrate. So we see that self-control is attainable, and the more we work at it, the more skilled we will become at using it when we need it.

This is just one of the qualities to me that makes up the beauty in us, that makes us unique, strong, and equips us to go on to the next phase in our lives. Everybody will not tap into this thing called self-control, but you can. Because I'm now telling you how I did it, how I lost my weight, and how I'm keeping it off. And I am certainly hoping that you can glean enough from all of my mistakes, disappointments and hurts. I would like to help you realize that if I could still do it (lose the weight) then so can you. If you really want to know how I did it, how I dropped 83 pounds and counting, then you should remember all that you have just read. Maybe you can find a way to keep it in your memory. Perhaps you can put it on your refrigerator, or in your bathroom. As long as you can see it, and remember the steps that I took to get to where I am today with this weight loss thing. Again I say, if I can do it then so can you. You can possess that great quality called self-control. Remember what I said, as you lose the weight, beauty is already in you, your job is to identify it, tap into it, and then master it. You know yourself and what you are capable of doing. Self-control is not to be taken lightly, and should be one of the things at the top of your weight loss list.

Another beautiful thing about us is that we possess this thing called will power. A very much forgotten attribute today, because of so many other ways to get you to where you want to be. I mean, why use your will power when you can just go to the store and buy certain things and don't have to resist anything. Why sweat if we don't have to, but that's a good band-aid if that is what you choose to do. But the greater beauty in that is, to use what you naturally possess to assure staying in control – because if something becomes a part of you then you have a better chance of it continuing throughout the long haul. Will power will take you a long way, your sheer will alone can cause a lot of things in your life to come to pass. For an example, if you wanted to lose your weight in a certain amount of time, and you put your mind to it, and acting only when you want to act. In other words, the more effort you put into it, the quicker you will obtain results from your actions. Eating only when you want to, and after learning about the things that would nourish your body. You are now armed with the information that's going to get you your results. So you activate your will power, and choose what and when you are going to eat. Will power is not something that's going to activate quickly. You might have to work at it, meaning you are going to make mistakes at the beginning but as long as you pick yourself back up, and keep on going toward your goals, in spite of the fall, then you should be okay. Will power is an asset to put in your armory of weapons in order to win the weight loss battle. Simple because it works together with everything else. What is hope if you have no will power to carry out the vision you are hoping for or what is self-control if you are not willing to carry out the orders that you have already learned to control. If we plan to use this thing called will power, then we must remember to generate it by knowing what we want, and what foods are not good for us. In other words, first educate ourselves on certain foods and then begin to think thoughts of self-control, where we can control our own thoughts to the degree our will power can be ushered in.

We have the free power to choose what we want to do, whether it is good of whether it is evil. I say power because it enables us to do something we would not ordinarily be able to do, whatever way you choose, in anything that's the way you want it to go. Whether it goes that way or not, it was your choice, you made your choice and whatever the outcome, you have to face the consequences. This also applies to our weight loss situation. We have the power or the right given to us to choose whether we want to put forth the effort to lose the weight. Taking myself for an example, for years I chose to keep the weight on in a round about way. I could have kept on pushing until I got what I wanted, but I chose to give up. I allowed hopelessness in and I gave up. But that was done out of ignorance. I didn't have the information I have now, the will power or the self-control. But now I know losing weight is an uphill battle that it's not going to happen overnight or easy for most of us. I can look back and say that it all made up a nucleus of me that would not have ever been made if I would not have gone through those ignorant times in my life. Those were the times that help build my character, the times that have brought me to these days of gladness and have kept me strong. Those were also the times in my life that have made me able to bask in my beauty, some things may have been disappointing and may have been ugly but I am picking up myself every day and keeping on until I fully conquer what I want to do, weight loss wise but that will only be a part of what I am going to accomplish because I just keep on pushing past the next storm in my life until I win that battle too.

If you look back at your weight loss blunders and think that it was all a mistake, you couldn't be further from the truth. Those are just things that you should remember not to do the next time; things to build you up for the long haul, things to add to your character and to your beauty.

Another key factor in weight loss is determination because after you have kept hope alive, mastered self-control, and tapped into your will power, then you are definitely going to need determination. You are going to have to be determined that no matter what kind of winds blow against your weight loss process, that you're going to maintain all that you have done. Some of us may have something in our life to go through that may be more detrimental than for others. This may be something that can cause you to pull out the fried chicken, the saltshakers and everything you resisted for years, but you have got to allow determination to keep you sustained. Because if you are determined, then no matter what comes your way, you won't allow whatever the dilemma is to give you a setback. It can come up against you time and time again but you are going to have to refuse to give in.

Your determination is going to make a world of difference in whether you keep going or not, in whether you throw in the towel or not. The question is how determined are you to get your weight loss issue under control? Establish your thinking right now because if you establish your thinking before the battle begins, then you can't do anything but win the prize. It may be difficult, but every pound you want to lose can be lost. I don't care how much you weigh, the weight can come off. But remember what I said, that only you can do it. Nobody else can do it for you. There is no quick fix to your weight loss situation. You're going to have to sweat it out. Also, don't lose weight for anyone else, lose weight for yourself only and remember not to worry about your past mistakes, they were all a part of the plan for your success. If you want to see beauty in action, then you might want to look in the mirror, because after you have heard these words of encouragement, I know that you have gone to the next level in this weight loss thing and that you are finally ready to bask in your beauty. You may not have made the step of putting down the fried food, red meat or the saltshaker yet, but you are ready to make a move. You are ready to possess those qualities that are going to get you to the next level. Your mind is getting ready to win everything you have been waiting for. You are now willing to make the necessary sacrifices and build yourself up with all the things that are going to help you get your weight loss issue under control.

Hopefully you are ready to bask in who you are going to be; who you are preparing yourself to be. Your mind is focused on thing but successfully accomplishing your weight loss task and a restoration you thought you could never have again. And remember, whether you are a man, woman, boy or girl, you are still beautiful and have all rights to obtaining any goal you want.

CHAPTER 5

Getting the Inner Healing
(While Getting The Outer Healing)

When we talk about an inner healing, we are talking about something that is very seldom discussed. Because on the inside of you is a part that feels, thinks, meditates, and harbors good things as well as what some might consider bad things. This is the part of you that makes you who you are. It stores information that only God and you can know. For instance, you might tell me one thing but on the inside you feel totally different. This is what I mean by things only God and you can know. People have been known to keep secrets 10, 20, or 30 years, sometimes even more. Whatever the secret might be may eat them alive every day, but if they are determined to keep whatever they know hidden, then most of the time there is not much someone else can do about it. This inner part of you is special. It forces you into who you are. You, at this point, may be saying, what does any of this have to do with losing weight. It has everything to do with it; you may have been picked on about your weight problem for years. Sometimes what people have said to you affects you so much that you tend to become what they said you are, whether what they said was good or bad. We sometimes transform on the inside into what that person said to us. For an example, if from your childhood you have been called ugly, fat, shorty or any other negative thing, you may now view yourself as ugly, short or fat even though this may not be your case. If someone likes one thing and they don't see that thing in you, then they sometimes make you feel like you're not living up to their expectations. When it's really your expectations you should really be living up to. Then you allow what others think about you to affect you negatively. Your self-esteem begins to lower. You become exactly what you said you would not because you have been pounded with the same thing continuously by several different people. You become infected with their thoughts of you. This is why I entitled this chapter getting your inner healing. Surprisingly enough, what you feel on the inside can determine how well you diet, how well you keep the weight off, and how determined you really are to conquer your weight loss issue. If you're always low feeling and tired, it's kind of difficult to muster up a whole lot of energy, physically as well as mentally to accomplish what you are setting out to do concerning losing your weight. Losing weight is strenuous at times, especially at the beginning. This is considered a crucial time. These are the times that you are either going to make it through the rest of your days of struggle or you are not. Your mental state at the beginning will carry you a long way. If your mind is not cluttered with other things, and it is somewhat clear, then you now have a chance to complete what you are trying to do. But as you go on in this weight loss thing, you will begin to see that you are going to need everything available to you to carry out your task. Your inner being plays a big part because it is the foundation of everything that you are about to do. It has to be healthy. Old memories of being called names, feeling left out of activities or employment because of your weight problem, or even people talking about you behind your back concerning your weight problem can hurt and affect how well and how fast you lose the weight. When this occurs to most of us; name-calling, neglect, overlooking for positions, can't get the date you want because you are considered overweight. It seems to sometimes damage what we call our ego, or our elf esteem because just when we thought we bought the prettiest dress in the store or got the nicest hair cut around, here comes someone to pull down everything that we have built up. Some of these insults may have been embedded in us for years, this means that the part of you that needs to be healthy is not healthy, but is full of those things that will not help you get to the next level in this weight loss thing. Losing weight demands your concentration, and if every time you go to take a run or a walk around the block and a flood of negative thinking springs up, for instance when someone told you that you might as well give up trying, you know that you can't walk past the first block. Also if you try to give up fried foods or change your diet and someone says you know you can't stop eating that fried chicken, I don't even see why you're trying. These are the unhealthy thoughts that have to be dispelled from your thinking. For a long time I suffered the teasing, the talks behind the back and the insults, but I took each and every one of them in stride simply because I had no choice. It seems as though when you ask a person to stop teasing because they are hurting your feelings, they may stop for a while but always seem to get back to your weight problem. Someone else begins to tease and joke about your weight, no matter what you feel. These attacks on your emotions can hurt you so much that you begin to believe them and begin to transform into what the people say that you are. Because if you hear you're too fat, you're too fat, you're too fat long enough, it begins to grow in you.

I say I took things in stride because you sometimes can't control what others do, but you must control what you do. So there I was hurting, offended, feeling trapped by the weight, discouraged and ready to give up. And I did give up on several different occasions. It took all that I had in me to withstand the hurtful words, the looks, the snickering, but I survived it and you can too. One of the main reasons I survived it was because after a while I somehow got the strength to ignore their ignorance and their disgusting remarks. I still say that it didn't happen overnight, it happened gradually, as time went on. It was either I was going to sink or swim, live or die on the inside and I chose to live. This is a difficult pill to swallow, especially when it may be someone close to you, someone claiming they love and care about you. But I say the same thing again, that if I can do it, you can do it. It wasn't easy, I went through changes as I said at the beginning, but I got past everything they said about me.

I now realize that I could have done something about the problem when the doctors advised me, but I chose to do what I wanted to do and the overweight problem was the consequence I had to pay. The constant weight gain and the injuries were still having a very significant part in my life, as well as, the tiredness and the shortness of breath. Just think, I could have saved myself years of this kind of self inflicted abuse and lived a much healthier life. But, as some people say, always learn from your mistakes. Maybe this could be you as the reader, someone that has injuries, and the doctor has advised you to lose weight, but you are choosing to do what you want to do. Remember my dilemma, if nothing else. I strongly suggest that you purpose it in your mind not to go through your life inflicted and abusing yourself as I did. Even with the hurtful things people said about me concerning my weight, this was enough to make me never surface in society again, but as I said, I got over the hurt and the pain by training my mind to ignore the statements and the ignorance of others. You may say to yourself, I can't do that, too much has happened; there is no hope that I will ever talk to those certain people again. But there is hope and it's up to you how far you allow things to go or how long you allow them to hurt because of their comments. If you want to know the truth about it, you are only hindering yourself. The same time and energy you are spending being upset with others can be spent developing a weight loss plan; seeing how you can get the weight off, what measures you have to take, where can you go to start your walking, and talking to your physician. These are very important steps to take, you have to have a beginning, and you must take time with yourself and plan things out. Even at the beginning if you don't have any money, you still can start right where you are. You may not have gym money or diet pill money, but you can walk, exercise, slack up on the portions of your meals, change your diet, and eat healthier. All you need to do is change your mind from what you don't have to what you do have. If you think about it, the things I just mentioned will not even cost you a dime. The only things you are going to need are a change of mind, will power, determination, common sense and a whole lot of hope. That is why being healed on the inside is so very important, because everything that happens has to come from you and you have to be willing to resist tempting foods, you have to have patience, keep hope alive and be willing to go on no matter what.

Your inner healing can take place when you begin to take control of the thoughts in your mind that have been dominating your thinking. Find a way to settle up with those deep wounds that have been placed there by others. The wounds that have crushed the trust that has been broken in past relationships and all the damage that has been done can be healed. It's going to begin with you, in your heart and in your mind. Forget about the past hurts, ignore ignorant people who do not have a clue to what's happening in your life. Moving into a better frame of mind can be done, if you just put forth the effort to do it, by changing your own thinking. You will know when you are healed because what people say won't matter to you anymore. You hear what they say and don't hear what they say. Your self-esteem begins to build, you think more of yourself, and you put up standards in your life that you have never put up before. For an example, if you are not losing weight fast enough for someone and they insist on calling you names, you now have the courage to walk away from them instead of argue with them, or tell them nicely, I beg your pardon, I'm losing weight and I'm not that same person that you knew in the past. Your confidence builds, you speak up, because you see how much work you are pouring into what you are doing and you will not allow anyone to stand in your way again. The control now is within you, like it was all of the time but you have now activated it. It seems like there's something about losing weight that puts you back in charge of your life, of your eating habits and of yourself. As you relieve your inner healing and get past those negative comments possibly embedded in your mind, said to you by other people, then you can make it. Even though before you began, you thought you couldn't. Isn't it nice to know that if you push yourself past the norm then you can accomplish what you are setting out to do? This is only being said to you in a positive and not in any harmful way; meaning, don't take what I have just said to do harm but only to do good. Life is indeed what we make it, and if we want to lose the weight successfully, and keep it off, then we may have some hills to climb, but it definitely can be done. As far as our inner healing goes, all we have to do is assert ourselves and we can be healed. We must not allow bitterness and anger to be a part of us, if we want to get what we need out of this weight loss thing. We have to do it in a way that we can see results and if it means that you have to go through your past and find out what's buried there so that you can deal with it and begin to work on a healthier inner you, then that's what you might just have to do.

Weight loss is serious and should be handled in a proper way. In your quest to lose your extra pounds, you should take it lightly, but make sure that you are tackling everything that you need to tackle to ensure that you are whole. What does it mean if you lose the weight and still hurt or feel depressed or discouraged all of the time? You are better than that, you deserve to be healthy mentally and physically and as long as you go day after day not dealing with the hurts and pains, then you are not all the way whole. I realize that it may take more for one than it might take for others, some may need to seek more in depth help but you can still be healed on the inside as long as you stick with it and allow yourself to take things day by day.

So, as this chapter comes to its conclusion, I'd like to remind you to believe in yourself. Believe that you can lose the weight you're trying to lose. See yourself in whatever size you want to wear. I don't care if it was 20 years ago; hold on to what you want. Remember I was a size 22, weighing 232 pounds and counting that may not be a lot to some but it was a lot to me. I can't even express how much better I feel since I first started losing the weight. It started for me a year ago; I started with the mind that I was going to fit a size 7/8 dress again. I was determined that the weight loss was just the beginning, that I needed my self esteem back as well. Along with forgiving the people who talked, laughed and whispered behind my back. At this time in my life, I can truly say that I have forgiven them, and that I have moved on with my life. If I could share this with you briefly, the same people that talked, whispered and laughed are now coming to me ranting and raving about how good I look and how much weight I've lost and how proud they are of me.

So, I'd like to leave you with these 4 words, just hang in there.

CHAPTER 6

The Finished Product

After my previous writings concerning your weight loss, at some point you should become the finished product. Once you have started the process of losing weight, you should be able to move from phase to phase. These phases are taken in stride day by day. I say in stride because you need not be in a hurry to drop weight that you have carried for the last 5, 10, 15, or 20 years. The object of the weight loss process is to learn as you go along, be aware of your mistakes and of your good qualities, as well as bad. You may want to learn and train yourself all over again. In fact, this is one of the moves I had to make in order to accomplish my goals because everything I did took a retraining. My mind had to think differently. Instead of eating fried foods all of the time, I had to train my mind to overlook the fact that stewed, baked or grilled wasn't exactly the way I like my food cooked but I had to do this in order to meet my goals. In the beginning I thought I could never do this, that this was for someone with a disciplined life. But as I continued to change my way of eating and as I grew accustomed to the change, I started making up recipes of my own. I began to experiment with foods and see what tastes better with what, what didn't look so appetizing or taste so good but I started enjoying these foods that I never dreamed I would even go near. It became a part of me.

Here I am, changing my foods after years and years of habitually eating one way. It was amazing. It kind of reminded me of the teachings given out in grade school, about the food groups and so on. I hadn't thought about that type of thing for years. Now I see that we are able to go back to what we already knew. If you noticed, almost everything

I told you from the beginning of this book until now, I already knew. I was already advised and warned. These types of things are evidently already embedded into our memories because it was years ago that I was advised by a physician to lose weight and it has been years since I heard the older fold tell me what to do and what not to do concerning weight loss. I don't even want to count the years that it has been since I learned about the food groups. So a change can happen if you will just find a way to change your mind, and turn your thinking around to making sure you accomplish what you set out to do. Don't give up no matter what.

The way to becoming the finished product is to complete the entire weight loss task; you cannot enjoy the fullness of losing the weight if you allow the weight to bring your wagon down. The weight of losing weight can be a heavy task in itself. It can bring your wagon down if you are carrying an extra load that will interfere with your weight loss process. For example, some of these loads can be finances, domestic problems, career problems, or anything that will hinder you from losing the weight. But whatever your situation is, if you work at it enough, it can be resolved. It does not have to be a weight or a load to what you are doing concerning your weight loss. Remember the old saying, it was the weight that broke the wagon down and you hopefully don't want to be a broken down wagon. We are still talking about the finished product, a person who has completed the, I'm going to lose this weight no matter what course.

So, after you have resolved your situations, then it's time to move on to another phase, as you can see, this is not a quick fix type of thing. This is a slowly roasted type of thing. You want to be slowly roasted because you don't ever want to go back to eating out of control and allowing your self to become overweight again. You want to be assured that you are in a clear-headed state when you do whatever you do. Even if you eat the wrong foods again, there is no one to blame but yourself because you have been slow roasted and everything that you are supposed to do is already grounded inside of you. Because you have learned about the long slow road and do not have to give in to temptation no matter what. This means you can hold on to the new you if you really want to.

If you choose to go against what you have already accomplished, then what you have already done, weight loss wise, is evidently in vain. You don't know if you will ever gather the courage to lose the weight again. Why take that chance? But once you've gone through the slow roasting process, then that should make a big difference in how you come through every test. You can supercede your goals and you can do better than you ever thought you could do.

The finished product is a superceder and a product that can stand the test of time. Standing the test of time doesn't always mean that it has to be something negative, it could be that you went on in your weight loss over a period of years, but even though you may have taken longer than others, for whatever reason, you should commend yourself also because you could not have been slowly roasted enough to go on in this weight loss thing to survive. Remember, this is something that you have to continue for a lifetime. My biggest warning is, do not lose the weight and think that everything is over. You have to make things a daily practice still. There will always be those old foods that want to draw you back. That's why you had to be slow roasted so that resisting those foods will be inside of you. Not that you are always going to be a superwoman or a wonder man but strongly believe that after you have done what you have wanted, weight loss wise, then you should reward yourself every blue moon with something special to eat, but that may not be good for everyone if you know that you are still out of control. Then maybe this is not the method for you. Or if your character is such that whatever you do, you are excessive and can't stop anything when you start, then you may not need to try the reward phase. Hopefully it'll be for another time.

The finished product is also able to withstand, even when the foods are still drawing them, they will either walk away somewhat hesitantly, or just plain turn it down. They may really want whatever it is. This means they have activated their will power and become determined that they are going to stay under control and keep up the good work. This finished product has definitely moved to another phase in their weight loss adventure. They have become so accustomed to making the necessary sacrifices that it is grounded in them to resist. Therefore, they know what they want and how much they want to do. They recognize their limitations and purposes in their heart to still maintain themselves in spite of what their appetite really desires. So to this particular person, I salute you and encourage you to keep up the good work because I realize that you have come over many hurdles. I remember that by the time I had come to this phase, it had become just a little bit easier for me also to resist certain foods, things, places and people. Believe it or not, this was my past time, dining out, sometimes being in the company of people that teased or insulted me. Of course, they said it in a joking way but as I would tell anyone, words hurt and at times they hurt me so much until they had me in tears. But I thank God that I have grown from hurting all of the time. I am at the point that I'm not concerned with what people say about me anymore. I'm still going on with my life and will continue to conquer those things that want to elude me. I am so confident because after I lost the weight, I took on a new attitude. My self-esteem is no longer low but I now see that I can do anything that I want if I really try. This also is evidence of a finished product because some people can hurt you so badly from what they say that you never recover. You never regain your self-esteem, confidence of anything else. The finished product is not fragile anymore, you may hurt a little bit, but you are able to shake if off before whatever the comment is totally affects anything about you. You are matured in this area, and more apt to continue the weight loss quest.

As I said, losing weight is serious and should be taken seriously. In order to achieve your weight loss goals, you have to become serious about it. Whether you have to rearrange your schedule, spend less time on the telephone, take extra time in the morning or evening for yourself. You have to find a way to become serious about what you are doing. It does not benefit you to, at first, do a lot to lose the weight and right in the middle, when you were about to go to the next phase, you fall apart. It may not be easy but no one knows you like you know yourself. Therefore, you know what it's going to take to cause you to take on a serious attitude about your weight loss issues. A finished product must be complete in every aspect. They can no longer afford to be slack in any area. It's too easy to fall back into the weight gain trap after a few times of slipping and sliding with your diet change, with your exercising and with your walking or running. We must stay on our P's and Q's at all times if we plan on losing the weight we said we were going to lose. You may now be asking the question, what scale is she using, how is she judging and determining who is the finished product and who is not. Well, if you really must know, I am writing from experienced knowledge. A knowledge that I have obtained from having to pass all the tests myself before I went on to my next phase. Everything I'm telling you at this time, I have been there and done that. This is why I can say that I realize that it's not going to be easy for some, because it wasn't easy for me. I struggled with temptations, falling back into the same traps, I got lazy, I didn't want to walk or exercise. But my famous words are, if I can do it, then so can you. So continue to be encouraged and if at first you don't succeed, then try, try again. If you're like me on one of those times things are going to sink in and the next thing you know, your mind has become serious, you're putting forth more effort like you've never done before.

When you used to fall off the wagon, your picking yourself back up, dusting yourself off and keep on keeping on. These are also good signs of a Finished Product. They may not seem to mean much at first but, as you go along, you will find out that every little thing, I mean the smallest thing you do in this weight loss thing matters. It matters how much effort you put forth because it determines how much weight you lose and how fast you lose it. And if you think a better attitude and a positive self-esteem don't matter in this thing, then you are definitely mistaken. Everything about you matters and adds up to the Finished Product I have been discussing with you in this chapter. Know that when you are finished, you can look back and say, I remember when I used to do that or didn't do that and be willing and able to tell someone else what you did to overcome those certain obstacles in their lives that have been keeping them captive. And wouldn't that be great, your weight loss spilled over onto someone else who desperately needs to hear a word of encouragement. It may be an aunt, an uncle, a sick grandmother, or even your mother. So as you go about your everyday living, and as you lose the weight, don't be surprised at who might be watching, and what their comments just might be. All of a sudden they may ask for your assistance in some area. They might need what you have for health reasons and so forth. So the Finished Product is always ready to answer questions and help someone else who has been struggling with the same thing.

If we take a closer look at the Finished Product, and if they looked in the mirror themselves, they probably would see where they used to be and what they used to be like, and that's good because hopefully, they will begin to see any other improvements that might need to be made. They just might look and say, I wonder how I would look with a shorter haircut, or I always wanted longer hair; I wonder how long it will take to grow to a certain length. Or, can I learn how to take care of my skin better, or my nails better? What can I do to add on to or enhance my weight loss? Will I get contact lenses or a new pair of glasses?

The Finished Product is always going to be searching for another way to better themselves and bring up his or her self-image. Looking in the mirror always seems to tell you a whole lot. It lets you know who you really are, not who you pretend to be or who you want to be, but who you really are and what you need to do for your betterment. Of course there may be cases that when you look in the mirror, you think thoughts that are not right but you can always overcome them if you want to. When you are a Finished Product, everything about you should begin to change, even those things that your physician told you just might come true. You just might begin to breathe better, you just might be able to walk up stairs, or some of your other ailments might begin to ease up. But I guess you, as the reader, will never know unless you try. I already know the truth about the advice I had been given, and now it's up to you. Whether you continue on the same way, or if you will just give yourself a chance. The choice is definitely yours and if by reading this chapter you have not come to the conclusion what the Finished Product is, then please allow me to explain it all to you so that you can know for yourself how important it is to be that Finished Product.

A Finished Product is one that has met all the necessary requirements and that product is now safe and fit to be open for display. But before that product was ready to go on display, or has been approved, it must first go through phases and processes. It works the same way for this weight loss thing, we must be ready for people to see us and say good things for a change, not things that will hurt and vex us. We deserve better than that. We should be called by our own names, not fatso or big mamma, etc. Another aspect of the Finished Product is that in order for you to be finished, you have to first make a start. You have to make a quality decision that I'm going to lose this weight, no matter if I have to run, walk, exercise, whatever I have to do to lose this weight that is exactly what I'm going to do. And, after you make your steps toward losing the weight you must remember that some things don't happen overnight and once again, give yourself a chance. If you're not satisfied with the way things are going, then get back on your horse and ride it again and again and again until you get it right. Believe it or not, you can get it right. The Finished Product has completed and successfully passed all the tests put before them and realize exactly what they have to do to keep the weight off. They know that it's going to be days when they are going to want to go on eating binges, that they are going to get lazy and don't do what they need to do in order to keep their physical body where it needs to be. So the main thing I can say concerning the Finished Product is, that they are quipped to get through the hard places and they know if they do something out of order, that they can get back in place and start again. Their mind is set to the fact that, I'm going to do this thing no matter what. When you become The Finished Product, you will confident in everything you have experienced during your weight loss battle. When things happen to make you fall off the wagon, you know that you have as choices to what you should do. It could be the death of a loved one, a marriage separation, a sick child, lonely nights, anything detrimental to you can trigger The Finished Product to feel that they can't go on, but they know that after they have lost the weight, took on a new attitude, built up their self image and scratched their way to where they are, then why lose it all now. As I said several times already, don't stay where you are, get back up on your horse and ride again until you get it right. As for the Finished Product, they also know that they are equipped for whatever may come their way because they took the time and lost the weight at a decent pace and found out that it's not about how fast you lose the weight that makes you successful losing it but it's all about being sustained after you have lost the weight. They are not eating the way that they were, they are not lazy about their body anymore because certain things are planted in them as they are going along and losing the weight in a good and safe way.

So, to all of you Finished Products, I take my hat off to you, and desire nothing but the best for you and yours, so stay encouraged and always look to find something else to repair and make better about yourself.

CHAPTER 7

Keeping the Focus

In this chapter I would like to share an important time in my life with you; when I first began to lose weight. That was a time I thought the most about giving up my weight loss battle, believe it or not. When I first confessed that the weight was coming off it seemed like everything I could think of began to happen. If it wasn't a problem with this, then it was a problem with that. These were things that demanded my attention and at that time, I did not have as much insight as I do now. I fell for some of the things I probably should have kicked to the side. My time began to be taken up with other things. I may have stayed on the telephone longer than expected then been too tired or too sleepy to exercise, or maybe it was too late to eat my last meal of the day. Whatever the distraction was, I fell for it almost every time, hook, lone and sinker. I found myself not home at certain times when I could have been there doing something to get me to the next phase of this weight loss thing. Disciplining yourself to things at a particular time can sometimes help you to carry out whatever your task may be. All this to say that at the beginning, it was very difficult to keep my focus. It was hard for me to keep my mind on what I was doing because I had so many other things going on. It became an inner war as to whether I was going to exercise or not. And this was almost immediately after I made my quality decision, saying yes, I'm going to lose this weight, even looked in the mirror several times and said it. But it seemed like the more I said it, the more I wasn't saying anything, almost as if I was just playing games with myself again. But little did I know that what I was saying in the mirror and to myself during the course of the day was seeping into my heart. I really meant it when I said it, but my actions dictated something else. This began to concern me; how can I say something and mean it but still do the opposite. But the concern that rose up in me was good, because I needed to push myself just a little more. I needed to put my actions where my mouth was. As I continued day by day, still sometimes struggling with doing the right thing to get my weight issue resolved, I realized that if I'm not going to accomplish my goal with this weight loss thing, I might as well go back to doing what I want to do. Not that I was getting that far, but at least I had started. As you well know, starting is okay, but it is whether you complete the task or not that is the most profitable. So, inch-by-inch, time after time, I started dealing with the distractions. I started making a conscious effort to look past the distractions. But in order for me to do that, I had to begin to watch every move I was making, not anyone else but I had to be conscious of things I hadn't thought about. Whether I was up early enough, whether I had enough rest, what times did I prefer to exercise, what foods did I really like the best, where were my favorite places to walk, was it safe enough; these were the questions. I had to ask myself these questions in order to pull myself out of the rut of allowing distractions to dominate my life.

This was a major step for me because I had always allowed distractions to take over, but never realized it until this certain time. Here was a perfect opportunity to change a character flaw about myself. It wasn't easy admitting that I was allowing sometimes petty things to have control of my day. But I took the challenge and started correcting things that made me lazy when I could have taken a walk, or eat fried foods when I knew that this wasn't helping my cause. These were just some of the things that were causing me to stay slowed down and hindered. Not even mentioning still associating with people who were not on the same mission that I was. This kept me distracted as well, and caused me to be influenced by still going to eat in restaurants and eating what I wanted. I was still out of control but as I said, I began to correct the things that were going to stop me from reaching my goals. It did not happen quickly, even after I made up my mind that I was going to change, it happened gradually. This gave another opportunity to be slow roasted and well-done concerning allowing distractions into my life. Each time I thought about things I had another conversation with myself. I became stronger in the distraction area. I took on a mind of; I'm not allowing distractions to be a part of my life anymore. Everything that even looks like it will disturb my focus in going to have to be dealt with and removed .It's not until this day that I realized the importance of keeping my focus in everything I do. I also learned so many other things that prompted me to move to the next level of my weight loss quest. But now I clearly see that your focus can mean everything to what you are trying to accomplish. When you are focusing your concentration is there, your mind can operate properly and succeed at accomplishing whatever you are trying to do. Focusing means you have a better chance at things turning out right, everything flowing in its proper timing but keeping your focus when things get tough can sometimes be very difficult. I realize that some things demand your attention and there is nothing you can do about it. But because there is nothing you can do but deal with the problem doesn't mean that your weight loss goals can't be met. It is possible to deal with more than one situation at a time. Some of us have the capability to solve several things at one time, so far those individuals, keeping the focus may not be a task but an adventure. Then there are those who do not keep the focus all they seem to know how to do is give their full attention to everything that comes down the pike. These are the ones that I would like to encourage at this time. I would like to just say you can keep your focus on your weight loss situation if you really want to. I'm not saying that to say this is all you should concentrate on. I know that other things are a part of life and that they also should be factored into your weight loss equations. When I first began this chapter, I spoke about the struggle I had with my focus and how it wasn't easy to do. But, if I could just mention to you that even though it wasn't easy, I ended up conquering that dragon too.

Another way I did it was tracking down where I was going wrong, what was hindering my flow? Once those things were located, I made up my mind that they had to be dealt with, and then even though it was still a struggle, I knew what had to be done. I took one thing at a time. When I found myself falling asleep and not exercising, I would change the time. Instead of trying to do it at night, I began to do it in the morning before I left the house. Another thing I did was, when I found myself slacking or turning back to my old ways, I immediately did the opposite of what I was doing. This helped a lot. I didn't allow things to escalate into a big monster so I would be unable to control it. Pinpointing things was a major strategy I used to keep my focus on my weight loss, as well as stopping things before they began. So you see, I did what I had to do to keep my focus on losing weight and also maintained every other thing in my life as well. Once I became skilled at pinpointing things, that was a definite victory for me because most of the time I really didn't pinpoint anything. The everyday things I did just seemed normal to me, not realizing that some of these very thing could become detrimental at another time, or that they could exist in my life so much, causing a problem in another area.

Keeping your focus is so important to your weight loss that if you don't keep it, you may not get too far accomplishing whatever your goals are. So, in light of that, I'm going to share a little more with you; how I did it, how I battled to keep my focus on my weight loss. I strongly encourage you to ask yourself questions such as; how are you going to keep your focus, and if your focus temporarily got off track what would you do to get it back? These are just a few of he questions that will help you put the pieces to your puzzle together. Your strategy has to be your strategy. You have to put things together to suit you and you only. As I mentioned to you earlier, in a previous chapter, there is no quick fix to this weight loss thing. You have to put it together piece by piece and day by day. You have to make your own plans as to how you are going to keep your focus, how you will put the pieces of your puzzle together, so that no one else can change it. This means you are going to be the one in control of how much weight you lose or how long it takes, or even how far you are going to go with this weight loss thing. As I go along, maybe you might want to think about your focus; where, what or who is it attached to? What is it going to take to get you detached? Remember your focus is going to get you over the hump and the more of it you have, the better. When I couldn't seem to keep my focus on my goals, I became discouraged and thought it was going to be like every other time I tried to lose weight, but there was something different about this time. I may have struggled, but I was still able to keep my focus enough to go to the next phase of my weight loss progress. Once I learned how important it was that my focus be fixed on my weight loss and how to keep up with it.

I had to continue to build my confidence level. I had tried to lose weight so many times before that it was a normal thing to give up and say I can't do this. I had grown accustomed to failing at it. But, instead of failing this time, I was succeeding; reaching goals and seeing inches and pounds drop off.

Needless to say, this was also a very exciting time for me but I must admit, a lot of other things came with the weight loss. One main thing was, it was now time to spend unexpected money. That means new pants, new blouses, new skirts, new dresses, because when the weight came off, that meant it was time for a new attitude. I don't know why spending these monies were unexpected to me. It should have been very much expected because after all, I was trying to lose weight. Maybe my focus was so much on losing the weight that I wasn't focusing on what was going to happen when the weight came off. This was in no way a negative unexpected thing but it was very much positive. It taught me that if you are expecting something, then expect everything else that goes with it.

Another thing that came with the weight loss was negative remarks. The remarks ranged from; are you sick, or is something wrong with you? Of course these comments were not welcome, but because people have the right to say what they want, especially when they catch you off guard, but the only thing that was important to me was still losing the weight. So my usual response was, no, I never felt better. This usually through them off because it definitely wasn't the answer they were expecting. So we see, to prepare for unexpected comments, once people visibly see the weight come off. But that's okay because you can survive that too, you can set yourself up right now for the negative remarks, for the unexpected finances to be spent. Some may have a little way to go, so if you have to save, then save. Or, if you want to take a leap of faith and buy the clothes size you want to be while you're losing the weight, then by all means do so. Whatever it takes to motivate you into keeping your confidence level up so that you can focus more on to the next phase, always be sure that you are comfortable while losing the weight. Being confident is what is going to help you to keep your focus where it needs to be and give you something to look forward to. It seems like there is nothing better than a good motivating tool to keep you going after you have worked yourself to the bone. You sometimes need something that is going to sustain everything that you have already done. As I said, whatever it takes to keep you going, I am in agreement with. Of course, this doesn't mean anything that can be harmful to you, such as unauthorized drugs. So, after you have stayed motivated, you are in a perfect position to complete your weight loss task. I realize that it's difficult losing weight and keeping our focus, so always have a reward at the end of your weight loss journey. Maybe that leap of faith dress or whatever you feel you deserve. But, if you don't remember anything I have said in this book, or if you have only read bits and pieces of it, of course I would like you to read, enjoy and learn from all of it, but I want you to remember to keep your focus. Expect the unexpected, lose the weight, and enjoy life. Those are going to be the moments you have been waiting for. They are to be treasured, embraced, cherished and appreciated.

In some cases you may have begun this weight loss thing with someone else as a partner, but they might have lost their focus but you must continue on. Celebrate yourself because you kept your focus, you stayed in the race, you conquered the dragons you needed to conquer, you win, Everything is now in your control, whether you keep up the good work and keep the weight off, or you allow yourself to skip back into an out of control state, it's all up to you. But don't forget what got you where you are; hard work, and that's what you have to continue to do in order to maintain everything you have done. The only thing now is that the work shouldn't be as hard. It should have gotten easier as time went on, you should have gotten used to exercising, eating differently, walking, resisting certain foods, controlling your thinking, keeping your hope alive and digging down deep inside yourself for strength so that you can succeed rather than fail. So that you can walk away with the prize, which is your new body, your new attitude, your new way of thinking. Forget about what happened before and start off new and fresh. Look for new ways to succeed with your weight loss whether it's getting a new career, etc. Because what happened before when you tried to lose weight doesn't even apply to now. Maybe you have gotten stronger in areas; maybe you've gained more wisdom in some things, and hopefully have received encouragement and insight from reading this book. I strongly ask that you don't be like myself, looking back; there was nothing to look back for. I had already failed, given up. There was no reason to ponder and focus on those things. Those thoughts were just a trap to keeping me thinking negatively and not positively. So that the only picture I saw would be failure, me not accomplishing anything concerning losing weight so just don't even try anymore, you're never going to lose anything so just forget about losing weight. Be fat, there's nothing wrong with you, you're healthy, you're eating every day, you have clothes on your back, food on your table, you'll find somebody that's going to take you just like you are. But even after all these thoughts, I still was discontented way down deep inside of me. I kept the weight on because I was naïve enough to believe that it couldn't be done. Even after prayer for years, but here I am, walking away with a prize many only hope for. You can be the same way; you can lose your weight as long as you keep your focus. I realize that some may be under the care of a physician and if that is your situation then I encourage you to continue as long as you are both satisfied. So, be encouraged, walk and exercise if you can do the things that can get you to where you would like to be in this weight loss thing. Because, as I said in a previous chapter, for some it could mean everything, your health, your very life. Weight loss is a matter of how well you keep your focus, meaning how much you do not allow negative thinking to control your weight loss goals. How much time will you invest in losing your weight, because if you are not focused you will not spend the time to work on your goals. Your focus at some times should be dominated by your weight loss goals but not obsessed.

So, as you and myself continue to meet our weight loss goals together, we must keep our focus because one of my main reasons for writing this book is to help you to get and keep your focus on whatever it will take to get you to meet your weight loss goals. Believe it or not, it can be done. We can get and keep our focus, achieve the goal, and snatch the prize. So again, I say be encouraged and don't forget you must keep your focus in order to get to where you want to be.

CHAPTER 8

How I Did It

In writing this book, I have made several different discoveries about myself, as well as, hopefully encouraged you, the reader. These discoveries were quite amazing when I thought about how long it took to lose the weight, and how long I had prayed to lose the weight, it totally took me by surprise, because it really didn't seem that long at all. I must have been extremely comfortable with my size, not realizing that these were years being taken off my life, carrying weight and having pain that no one should have had to bear. But even after all of this, how could I mentally stand the inward battle, the battle of, I really want this weight off but I'm tired of trying. That, I think was the most difficult thing to deal with, the fact that I wanted to do something about myself but couldn't overcome the battle of food. Food had no problem with me; I had the problem with food. I guess that just goes to show you that everybody who's in a bad or awkward situation does not always deliberately want to be there. So there I was, struggling, warring, battling and ultimately giving up to something that seemed to have a choke hold over my appetite, life and will. The discovery I made was that after all I had been through in trying to lose the weight, some of the things I did to get the weight off was just plain and simple. Of course it was difficult at first but once I got up and running, that was all I needed to take myself to the next phase. Losing weight was a new adventure every day. I began to think of different ways to do things. I thought about what the doctors told me to do and for once, I did it. This was simple after a while. All I had to do was remember what I was told in the past, not just by the doctors but also by other people. It was a shame that it took years to see the light, but at last the light has now been seen.

Another discovery that I made was that even though it took a little time to gain momentum, I saw that I was able to do something that had totally defeated me for years. This was good for me, that I was finally winning the battle. Just think, I probably could have won from the beginning if I would have pushed and pushed even if I fell off the wagon, got back up and started pushing again. But why cry over spilled milk, the point is, I have a major victory in my life and I am going to enjoy every minute of it. Those are the times to look back on and say, I didn't think I could at the beginning but look at me now. I made steps to look to a new phase in my life and it paid off. Making steps sometimes are not the easiest things to do because most of the time our minds are so cluttered we can't see the forest for the trees, let alone focus enough to make steps toward anything, but when I made my steps, I took one day at a time, just as some of you did who have conquered certain areas of your life.

Now you might want to take a closer look at what you can do next to enhance what you have already done concerning your weight loss, just as I did. Whether it's beautifying yourself, or picking out new outfits, whatever you see about yourself that you can do safely for your betterment. You might need to look into it because if you can do one thing that you thought you couldn't do, then you can do another. But to continue on, I'd like to also discuss my time of prayer; because this was definitely one prayer I was exhausted waiting to manifest. I must say that I never really gave up faith. Even though I gave up hope, I had to rely on someone that had what I needed, which was strength and hope, because mine was down to a bear minimum. I had given up but I see now, that was the thing to keep me alive as I keep the weight off. Hope is not something that you pull off of the shelf and put it back on, hope is something that you have to keep and cherish. Because of the fact that I lost my hope, I had to pick myself up from a pit that only God helped me crawl out of. Hope was a valuable asset to me as I went along, and not only in meeting my weight loss goals but in my everyday living. I thank God for His mercy, even in my time of hopelessness. And as I continue to share a little more about how I did it, how I did what so many other people have tried to do so many times and were unable to succeed.

What I simply must say is that how I lost the weight was not as important to me as what I gained as I lost the weight. I mean, it was quite interesting learning new things about myself, which, evidently were there all the time. Things that I could have done to make my life much easier, but chose another route. I say this because the things I gained were an elevation in my self-esteem, a battle I had for years and just could not seem to win. Maybe it was my childhood or maybe it was my environment that caused my self-esteem to be zero. I often didn't think much of the way I looked years ago. I didn't think I was the prettiest girl in town but not the ugliest either. As a matter of fact, I didn't really know what self-esteem was at that time. I either thought of myself one way or the other. Either I looked nice one day or I just considered myself to have a bad day another but I've learned through this weight loss thing that self-esteem is a very valuable tool to possess. It can determine how far you allow yourself to go in life. For example, if you don't esteem yourself highly, you just may not go on that job interview for that top-notch position in the company. You may not think that you qualify for whatever reason, whether it's your looks, your weight, or your lack of education. Whatever your particular hang-up might be, but self esteem will say, I'm going for this job, I'm just as qualified as anyone else, I look just as good as anyone else, and my credentials are as up to par as anyone else's. Even if I am not chosen, it wasn't because I didn't try or I didn't put my name on the list. So you see, it's all according to what we feel about ourselves that pushes us to the point of saying; I can do whatever I want to do in life. Everything I can think of, I can perform all of the time not part of the time. I am, of course, applying this to positive things, not hurtful or dangerous things. We are focusing on what is going to help you keep your life in order. Self-esteem is a major part of that; at least it was for me. Ironically enough, everything in a way has been good for me, even the weight because I might not ever have known how much I'm capable of doing. My self-esteem is at an all time high and I feel so well rounded. I'm also hoping that you would like to be a well-rounded person at this point, someone who not only wants to meet their weight loss goals, but also wants to know about the extras that come along with it. For me it was recognizing the strengths I didn't know I had, amongst other things, but for someone else they might gain self control, or learn better eating habits or take their doctor just a little more seriously when he or she gives them advice. This is not saying that your doctor is always right because I really don't know that. All I do know is, because you have to put so much into losing the weight, you might as well have it all. The weight loss, a new mind, a new attitude, everything you could possible have gotten out of it. Anything that will build you up is what you need.

Continuing in this chapter, let's consider everything that is at stake when you meet your weight loss goals. What I mean by, at stake, is at risk. If we don't prepare ourselves properly we will not survive the weight loss process. Our health, finances, time invested, and things we have done will be wasted, not withstanding when times get hard. For example, when you feel like eating in the middle of the night, or when a tragedy may befall you or your family, you may automatically turn back to food. If we would just learn while we are working on ourselves to think about the whole picture, then we will survive everything that will come our way. This is the way I had to train my mind to think as I went along. It became less difficult as I developed new ways of meeting my goals. My mind transformed into thinking about the future. Some of the questions I asked myself were; what am I going to do once I lose the weight, what has this all been about, am I losing the weight just to be losing it, or do I have a purpose in mind? I remember once saying to myself, this is a lot of work, and I wonder should I look into pursuing a career that's going to change my whole image. Something nobody ever expected me to do, so you see, there are other things to consider before, during and after we lose weight. These things may range from track, modeling, business owners, and so on. Whatever you envision for yourself can be done so I strongly urge you to think about what you really want to do. Is your weight hindering it, if you lose the weight, would it make a difference? Focus your thoughts on yourself and make major decisions because there is life after the fat and it's up to you how much you get of it before, during and after you lose the weight. Purpose it in your heart that once you meet your goals that you want to be well rounded. You want to finally be satisfied with you, that for once you're going to say, I am totally and thoroughly, 100% in control of my life. Whether I pursue another career or not, I'm satisfied with the way I look, with what I have done with myself and where I am going from here. Losing the weight was wonderful but there is more to me than to lose the weight. There always has been more to me than losing the weight and always will be. No matter how much they teased me, how much they talked about me, I have always been and will always be somebody. Now that I have accomplished this great victory in my life, I know that I can do whatever I want to do in life and maintain it without falling apart at the seams. Yes, this is a great time in your life because you have hopefully made the better choice of losing the weight and keeping yourself in good health. I am definitely hoping that this book has somewhat inspired and encouraged you to think about yourself in a whole new fresh way. Even if it's just caused you to meditate on what has already been told to you by doctors, friends, or family. At least this is a beginning, somewhere to move on from here. You can now take those thoughts and determine whether you want to take things further or you don't really want to invest your time and efforts into losing weight at this time. As I told you in a previous chapter, it really doesn't cost that much money or maybe no money to lose weight. I also told you that the choice is yours, you have the power of free choice, no one can twist your arm to do anything, especially something like this. Losing weight is for your own benefit, it can only help you in the long run and as I also said, you have to lose weight for you and only you. You have to be satisfied with you and willing to change whatever it is you have to change to go to the next phases of your life. It took me a long time to learn that I had to lose weight for me because it didn't seem to mater whether anyone pushed me or not. I had to put forth the effort. The effort had to come from me. I had to put my best foot forward and take on the dragons that were stopping me from losing weight. That was when I got victory over the eating problem, the low self-esteem, the not looking my best. When I overcame these things, even thought it wasn't the easiest thing in the world, it seemed as though I somehow received a new strength to defeat the next dragon I had to defeat.

I got knocked down, discouraged, made mistakes but I picked myself up and grew in something called determination because it seemed like all I needed to see was the inches come off, the pounds drop off, and my dress, pants and blouse size changing. That's when I knew I was on to something that wasn't impossible after all, that this weight loss thing could be done. It was my choice whether I kept on going or I stopped in mid-stream. I had to shake off the old ghost; nobody else could do it for me. The effort had to be put forth and it had to be put forth while I was in the mood. So I'd like to continue to encourage you at this time to make up your mind and then take steps toward your goal. Even if they are baby steps, and purpose in your heart not to stop no matter what. You may fall of the wagon, you may lose the schedule you may have put yourself on, but you can put it all back together and defeat the dragons in your life. Whether it is laziness, discouragement, giving up, hopelessness, or just plain don't care, everything is in your hands. You have to make the ultimate decision whether you are going to stay in whatever state you are in.

Let me remind you that I did it by hanging in there, by being patient and recognizing when I had the upper hand. Rejoicing and celebrating when I went from phase to phase, victory to victory. I had to rejoice when I saw the pounds dropping off and me looking like my old self again. This, of course, was the moment I had been waiting for. After years of seesawing, trying to lose weight, my time had finally come. My figure was coming back, as well as feeling like my youth was coming back. Suddenly I felt like a new person, someone that had been released from a terrible bondage and weight. I was getting my life back from all the things that had plagued me for so very long. It was a miracle and I was, and still am, basking in what has taken place in my life. As I said so many times in this book, it wasn't easy, but it has been done. If any of the people that talked, laughed or teased me in the past concerning the weight would dare to say anything to me today, it could only e how well I look and how did you do it? How did you take the weight off, and what have you done to yourself to look so doggone good? These are questions that I can answer with a smile on my face and say I did it with prayer, patience, determination, self-control, making positive choices, allowing my self-esteem to be built up, and working on myself every day. I allowed myself to change and transform into who I really am, the woman I missed out on for 18 years. A woman denying herself of certain privileges simply by not obeying medical and other advice, a woman who could have been slimmer and almost pain free for years. Instead of enjoying those years, I was overweight and hurting all of the time from the neck on down. I could have been a woman fulfilling her dreams, hopes and purposes in life. So now, I take the opportunity to recover all that I have lost during my period of ignorance. I have told myself that everybody makes mistakes and that I'm no exception to the rule. Meaning, just because I may have lost that time, or it appeared that I have lost that time, doesn't mean that things have to stay that way. This could have happened to anyone, so there is no need to blame myself or anyone else for my mistakes but continue to move on and make every minute precious and valuable. Other things I could tell someone when they ask me how I did it is changing the types of food that I ate, sometimes eating one meal a day, as well as ate fruits, nutritional drinks, no red meat, walking, working out and taking better care of myself, no sodas, very little sugar if any, little salt if any, no junk foods if any, few potatoes if any, no white bread, no seasoned fatty lunch meats, low salt only, no sugary candy, no hoagies or anything to that nature, no slacking up after a while. I also make a schedule of what I had to do every day, what time I wanted to do it and how long I was going to do it. For example, if I walked on the treadmill, I constantly increased my time and as the weight began to come off I walked on it even longer. I stretched my walk times to my limit but remember my limit may not be your limit so examine yourself and take note as to how long you can walk or run on the treadmill. You might want to discuss it with your physician just to make sure that this is the right thing for you, while you are losing the weight. You might want to make yourself a schedule; as to how long you can do whatever it is you want to do to determine your longevity. As I went along losing the weight, I substituted salt for sometime nothing, maybe used a salt substitute a few times, but that was it for the salt. I cut down on my fried foods, almost to none at all. I purposely stopped frying chicken, pork chops, hamburgers, steaks, and all the things I used to love eating and usually fixed, I brought to a crawl. I sacrificed day and night whether it was in the gym sweating, in the kitchen denying myself of my favorite foods, in the morning or at night, when I decided to walk and or exercise I sacrificed time that I used to do unimportant things to get the rest I so desperately needed. These are most of the things that I did to lose 83 pounds and counting. I did it without any drugs. I did it with very little money. I did it at a time when it wasn't the best time in my life, but I took the challenge and won the victory. So, if you really trace back to what I have been saying in this book, you can accomplish what you are setting out to do by simply observing that I didn't have everything to pull this off. I thought I should have had but I lost the weight anyway. It wasn't what I thought it should have been like, but I lost the weight anyway. So, if I can encourage you in any area, it would be to not look at your present situation and determine whether you should attempt to meet your weight loss goals, but to examine everything around you, pick your time, meaning a time when you can see yourself doing everything that you have to do to lose the weight. And I warn you that no time is going to be a good time, you are going to always have something you have to do. Somewhere you have to be, a reason why you can't run, skip or jump, no time in between the jobs, the husband and or the kids, so this leads me to tell you that you are going to have to take control by just doing it. Fix your schedule the best way you can and go for what you know. It may even seem that it will not work out but if you revise things according to your needs, everything should work out fine. As you put your plan together, watch out for booby traps where you might put something together and it never materialize into anything. Every time you go to do what you plan, something always comes up, or you don't have the place to do it, or it seems silly so you back off, but if you would hang in there, and expect the unexpected then when distractions and problems come, you can tip toe around them and make the best of a bad situation. You can accomplish your weight loss goals if you really try.

As I bring this chapter to a close, I certainly hope that you have gleaned something to take you to the next phase of your weight loss or have motivated you enough to say, I'm going to do what I have to do to lose this weight, and I'm not going to stop until I accomplish what I have set out to do, then I will know that the information you have received from me, as to how I lost the weight and went from a size 22 to a size 10 was effective and that you intend to take every bit of it seriously enough to put it into play in your life. Now that is a great feather in my cap.

CHAPTER 9

Keeping the Weight Off

If I could just have your attention for the next few minutes, it would definitely benefit you. I have discussed mostly methods on how to lose the weight, what you can do, how you can do it, and I hope that has been helpful and informative to you. In addition to talking to you about getting the weight off, I'd now like to discuss how to keep the weight off. If you remember when you first began to lose your weight, hopefully you have started, and things were rough at the beginning but you survived it all; the walking, even though your head and legs didn't always agree with each other, you still somehow managed to push yourself out of the door or when you wanted sleep and your conscience kept nagging at you to get up and exercise, or maybe you remember the body aches that came when you first began to walk, exercise or work out. I ask you to bring these memories back because these are the things that will help you along the way in this chapter. If you can remember all of the things which occurred when you first started, then hopefully you are saying to yourself that you don't ever want to go back to that stage of your weight loss again. Not many people survive the first few days, weeks or even months of exercising, walking, dieting or even working out. They often stop after the first couple of aches and the first time it seems as though things look like too much work. This is where some may have fallen off the wagon and never recovered. That is why that time period is so important, because it either makes you or breaks you. You either become grounded well enough to move on to your next phase or you stay there until you find a way to strengthen yourself. That stage cannot be avoided. Everyone has to experience that time of strengthening their will power, their mind and their emotions but the real purpose of this chapter is to keep you on your toes against anything that could possibly come your way to destroy your weight loss accomplishments. Every time you think you are strong in an area doesn't mean you are strong. You can easily slip into fast foods, fried food, over eating or into all kinds of high calorie desserts. It doesn't take long; you may not even notice yourself eating some of the children's snack, a little more than usual. As I wrote in a previous chapter, these aren't foods that you don't want; these are foods that you do want. These weren't foods I just wanted to give up, I had friend chicken a few times a week, if it wasn't that, it was fried pork chops, or whatever other food that satisfied my taste buds and I enjoyed eating them. I also fell back into them at times and wasted a lot of what I had already done. We weight watchers can't afford to think we are stronger than we are and deceive ourselves into thinking we can handle even a little of what we used to eat. We definitely do not want to go back into that time in our weight loss process of wasting our time again. I have kept my weight off now for over a year, and I still know that fried foods might not sit to long around me. I'm not foolish enough to think that I can't fall back again into that same rut. Even though I feel strong and confident in what I have done with myself, it took a while to build any confidence and I don't' want to lose that valuable asset called confidence, something we should possess if we want to meet our weight loss goals.

Guarding certain parts of our character is a must if we want to keep the weight off. Confidence, encouragement, motivation, determination, rejuvenation are just some of the valuable characteristics that we as weight watchers should have in order to maintain what we have already done. I use the word guard because these attributes have to be protected from the everyday incidents, trials and dilemmas that can easily take you away from your strategy. In order to survive the opposition, meaning the things that will interfere with what you are trying to do. You must protect everything about what you are doing by first recognizing your attributes. Are you determined to get what you are after, can you stand to be a little more motivated? How high is your confidence level, even if things don't go right, can you keep your confidence up enough to bounce back from difficult times and say I can still do this thing? I can still lose this weight. If you don't know what makes you tick then you are going to have a hard surviving when things get rough. You also will have to pull out the patience when you get frustrated and ready to quit, just like I had to do. Then when you feel like it may not be worth it, because of aches and pains, you're going to have to go back and remind yourself why you are doing this. Whether its for health reasons or you just want your appearance up to par, you are still going to have to have some kind of a way to get yourself back on track again. Maintaining your weight is a very important part of losing the weight itself. If you don't know how to keep it off, then you will probably gain it back over a period of time. As I wrote before, it is difficult at the beginning; attempting to lose the weight. You have worked hard and long. That is not a place we should want to go back to but if you should allow yourself to lose control of the weight again, you may not get another opportunity to lose the weight like you did this time. So, keep on going with whatever you know to do to keep your weight off. Also, in maintaining your weight, we must keep or have a certain degree of order so that we know what we have to do almost every second of the day. Even if you have to keep a journal, you need to have some form of structure daily, something that you do over and over again and should begin to come natural but for some, it may take a miracle. So, I want to help those who always seem to be doing something else when it's time to walk. I do realize that things happen to distract your day, but in that case, you just have to find your place again and keep on moving toward your goals. You may ask what does order or structure have to do with me losing weight. If you think about it, everything, because some readers may have children who need their attention or some may have a spouse who they have to attend to, or some may have a sick loved one who needs caring for. These are people who need not to be neglected, that is why you need order because you may have a full life already and squeezing exercising, diet changing, and working out into some of your lives may look impossible but it can be done as long as you have structure, good planning and use wisdom. You can plan everything out so well that you can get everything done that you want to get done with time to spare. So, remember that once you learn the skills of order, planning and structure, you already won half of the battle. That's how essential these three things are to keeping your weight off. You must not neglect or continuously put off your responsibilities to meet your weight loss goals. As with everything else, you prioritize and do first thing first. We also can keep our weight off by continuing to do the same thing we did to get the weight off. Just because we are the size we always wanted to be, we mustn't forget what got us there; hard work and sacrifice.

If we joined a spa, then we might want to keep working out. If you have tremendously changed your diets like I did, then you might want to think of new and better ways to cook your chicken, turkey or your fish. Even vegetables can be seasoned in such a way that they taste better than they ever tasted before. Keep your newly found ways, they are a part of staying alive when it comes to keeping you at whatever size you are. You may not take keeping the weight off as serious as taking the weight off but that is a critical mistake so many people make after they get to where they want to be. This is the reason for this chapter; to make sure that you are aware of the fact that this is a never ending adventure and to help you see just that. I want you to take everything seriously in this book and to know that there are ways to keep the weight off. Even if you have to get someone else to support what you are doing, by holding your hand through your hard times or maybe they just want to be there for you in case you need them. Whatever the need is at the time, they can be a major support for you if you pick the right person. Be sure they are someone you can trust and confide in, as well as have time for you when you need them. They may be able to encourage you when things get rough, or may go shopping with you as your sizes change. Just keep an open mind, meaning be selective, because it may not be a good idea to choose someone just because they may be close to you. They may not have patience, time or be compassionate enough. This does not mean that they are a bad person but that they just might not be right for what you need them to do. Explaining that to them would be a good idea so that the situation won't become a problem.

Another thing you might want to consider in keeping the weight off is making it fun. You may say how can I make this fun, I just sweated till I dropped, burned myself out, you still may be hurting in places you didn't know you had, but inside of you is still the capacity to enjoy yourself. Even after all you've been through, you have to remember that there is a part of you that wants to go back to the way you were weight wise. You must watch yourself in all areas while you are losing the weight because after the doctors have warned you, your family and friends teased you, you were sick of yourself. All this to say that you made your decision to lose the weight and came to the conclusion that it was time to change so that means don't be tricked into giving up all you have accomplished already, and because you now see that you could have lost the weight the whole time so you should want to make it fun and want all of the things that come with it. For example, if one of your desires is to go to the mall to the store where everybody could buy something but you, because you were overweight. Now just think, all you have to do is have the money to buy whatever you wanted from the beginning. Or remember when you didn't want to go to the family reunion because of your weight, or to the class reunion because what you wanted to wear just didn't look right in your size. Now you can go and smile with the same ones who teased, laughed and belittled you, with nothing in your heart negative about them and enjoy yourself. Hold your head up high, showing off what you've done and reaping all the benefit of your sweat and tears. So, we see that there is more to get out of this than just the weight loss. You can make it fun also by now doing things you couldn't do before you lost the weight, such as water ski, hiking, skating, bowling, whatever it was that excited you before you lost the weight can still be done. But again for some who are under doctor's care, please check with your physician. Always be safe and have peace of mind as you enjoy the things you have wanted so long to do. Make sure that you do not harm yourself in any way, this is why I say that it may be wise to consult your physician before doing anything that could affect your health.

We have now covered many bases as to how to keep the weight off, but I would also like to discuss getting used to yourself, changed, different, slimmer, where you want to be and looking to the future. In order for us to keep our weight off, we are going to have to like the finished product because after you win your weight loss prize, you just may not like who and what you have become. For the simple reason that other things in your life may not have changed as you were changing. Your clothes may look out dated, your hair may not be long enough now that you have lost the weight. Are you too skinny, can you get used to your thighs not rubbing together? There could be endless topics to discuss concerning whether you like the finished product or not. We will only talk about a few important issues that could turn you around and make you begin to overeat again. After you have lost the weight, take a good hard look at your masterpiece, which is going to be yourself. Are you satisfied with what you see? Can any other changes be made? This is your decision to make; you are going to have to like yourself in the morning. Keeping the weight off is a condition of the heart; you are going to have to be glad that you took the weight off. Sometimes being glad alone is going to encourage you enough to keep on working out, keep on running, walking, and finding new ways to eat your foods because if you are glad about something, you want to continue to be pleased by it. You are not going to want whatever it is to stop so whatever it is you are glad about should make you do whatever it is you have to do to keep it that way. If you are pleased with your self, and hopefully you are, then it will not matter what you have to do to keep the weight off, you are going to do it because you know that it is worth every bit of the sacrifices you are making to get to where you wanted to be. Therefore, you are going to continue in your good works and keep everything under your subjection. The reason I say that it is a condition of the heart is because it's according to what's in your heart, concerning yourself, that is going to make all of the difference in the world as to whether the weight loss stay or whether the weight loss goes. Even problems can cause you to view yourself negatively and allow things to seep into your heart while you end up saying, I'm tired of trying to keep control, I don't have time for this right now, or have to many other things on your mind and in your heart that weight loss is not your first priority. So, you ultimately end up forgetting about it and never getting back to it, or you just keep it in the back of your mind and still never get to it. Now we see that it is important to keep our minds and hearts clear, this is the best thing so that we can concentrate fully on our weight loss situation. We need every ounce of our concentration; this is why we have to continue and should not become stagnated. Once other things occur in our lives, we have to be able to maintain our stride in losing the weight and should not be in a position to waste valuable time. Be consistent, and make every day, minute and second count. Enjoy yourself, celebrate yourself, reward yourself, because the sad thing is that if you don't do these things for yourself, maybe nobody else will.

As we move to our next chapter, I'd like to leave you with these words of encouragement. Stand firm against the things that would come your way to hinder and to discourage. You can keep yourself strong by continuing on your same path because if it's working, why change it? Keep building yourself up and make it a point to use what you have built to keep fighting the opposing things in your life to keep your weight under your control. You can keep the weight off if you try.

CHAPTER 10

Doing It Right

We have discussed many subjects in this book, but the overall thing should be for us to do it right, as well as produce in this weight loss thing. Doing it right doesn't necessarily mean that you are going to do everything right every time. It means that you take your time as you go along and become cautious about things that you do. This can transform you from doing things that you want to do to things that will help your weight issue. Because there are certain things that you have to do in order for you to glean anything out of this book, you have to learn how to do it right first of all but I also realize that you are going to make your mistakes, but as I said before, you just pick yourself up from where you are and keep on moving. The reason why I am telling you as the reader, that you have to do things right is because you should want to be healthy as you lose weight. You want to be safe as you lose weight and don't overly exert yourself. Your thinking has to be where you need it to be, when you are losing weight. Your doctor should be informed as you lose weight, he or she may want to give you any instructions that should be specifically designed for you. This could range from what exercises to do or don't do, how long to walk, what you have to do to get the results that you want? Losing weight takes your concentration and a whole lot of will power. This is why I say that your mind has to be where you need it to be. Some things we take for granted in life, and for some of us it is our thinking. We must remember that our minds control so much about us, and we have to make sure that we take good care of it. If I had to say anything else about our minds concerning weight loss, it would be that keeping it focused on things that can help you get to the next phase of your weight loss task would be the best thing for it. I realize that's not easy, but it has to be done. This is part of you doing things right, keeping your focus, thinking about things that are going to help you, and concentrating fully on what you have to do with your weight loss. Things at home may happen, things at your place of employment may go wrong your life may be leaving you with issues to deal with but as you do it right, as far as keeping your focus, and your concentration in tact, you can attend to every last one of your situations and still keep your motor running for your weight loss. You can do this because of the time you have built up focusing and concentrating and also putting into action what you were thinking about, which should be nothing but positive thinking, which should bring about positive results. So, we see, our thinking has everything to do with doing things right. We even need our thinking to think to do things right. It is important to think right.

Another thing to consider while you are losing weight is to follow any instructions that you may be given whether it is from your doctor or anybody who may have any influence over what you are doing. Hopefully you have put yourself under someone's care who is professional and experienced in caring for your needs. If this should be the case, they should have no problem instructing you as to how to be safe, and how to do things right. Your medications should still be taken. If you have a certain disability, you still may want to pay close attention to your instructions so this is not something that you might want to run rampant with and do whatever comes to your mind. You should do things in an orderly fashion and make sure that you consider every need as you go along. Losing your weight is going to have to be done your way, as I said before. There is no quick fix, no one else is going to or can lose your weight for you. You are solely responsible to make sure that you do it right and that you dot every I and cross every T. I say this because you are the master of the ship, and whatever you do can mean everything. You may have been told by your physician that you shouldn't eat certain things or you can't bend or lift, or you could damage yourself even further, or that if you don't lose weight then certain unpleasant things could occur in your body, so you being the master or the captain of your ship has to know when too much of a certain thing is too much. You must remain in control and do things right. If you want your desired results, you also have to complete the things you begin. For example, if you have a series of exercises to do, given by an instructor, and you only complete half of your program, then you may not get your desired results in your weight loss. As for me, I basically did things on my own from past experiences. I could have obtained even better results if I were under professionally structured care. You always want the full affects of what you are going to do, which is lose the weight, so you want to complete everything instructed by your caregivers provided everything is in agreement between you and them. Doing things right can also include not eating foods that you know can be harmful to your health, even though you have acquired new taste buds. This could be something that you were allergic to before you began to lose the weight, which means that you are probably still allergic to it. Don't take chances, watch what you eat, and how much you eat, but of course you already know that. Being in control of your weight loss is important so as I said before, you have to lose the weight right. Right meaning, properly, so that you can look your best, feel your best and think your best. If you don't do it right, you may have labored in vain, your end result may not be exactly what you expected. For instance, if you have planted roses, you don't expect tulips to row at harvest time. This means in weight loss terms that in the end, you want to look like you've worked hard to look like, not feeling out of shape or have gotten sick or sicker from possibly not taking your medications, or so tired and burned out from walking, exercising or whatever you did, that you can't even enjoy your accomplishment. You simply must keep control and make sure that you are the master or captain of your ship. Working so hard to lose the weight will not even be a factor if you don't lose the weight right. Because when the pounds come off, the pants get bigger, the dresses don't fit anymore, you will probably look in the mirror and say, it was worth it all. The sacrifices, the times of having to be flexible to change things, the times when you didn't want to go on with it anymore, and you just wanted to give up. Even after it looked like you weren't getting any results, but you still hung in there and make sure you have done it right. You can see the finished product right in front of your very eyes. Someone slimmer, wiser, looking as good as they want to look. This is hopefully the results of someone that has done things right, someone who has taken precautions, who has made sure they are healthy, that they are thinking correctly and everything they have done thus far has been of their own accord. They've taken their meds. You are someone special, and have always been someone special, even when they teased you and hurt your feelings, you were even special then. You might not have realized it at the time, but if you look at yourself now and look at yourself then, I know you are going to see a very special person. Not just someone who has lost 50 or 60 pounds but someone who has also changed on the inside, someone who has hopefully forgiven those teasers, and backbiters, someone who has taken control of their life in more ways than one and has tapped into parts of themselves that they didn't even know they had. You are now your own finished product, and whether you like what you see in the mirror or not, you are now looking at who you have wanted to be for a long, long time. It's up to you what you do from here, and what you make come out of things. If you wanted to be a model or an actress, or a doctor or a lawyer, now may be your time to go for it and now that you have done things right, you can enjoy the fruits of your labor. You can enjoy the weight loss without being tired and looking sick, or worrying about what you have right or wrong during the whole time because the expected end result is now here and you are looking right at it. All because you have done things wisely, by losing the weight right, not a barrel of problems following you after you've reached your weight loss goals. Believe it or not, doing it right starts when you first begin to lose weight, a lot of people think you wait until the middle of your weight loss task but if you start at the beginning, that will definitely help in the long run. In case you have not caught on to what I mean by doing it right, and how I judge or say what is right or wrong, then you might want to look at your present state. If you are weight watcher, and have lost quite a bit of weight, over a period of time like I did, hopefully you now see yourself after you've lost the weight in a positive manner but for some they may have had difficulties. For instance, if they have lost more weight in certain parts of their body than in others they may some extra work to do to fully tone up. It seems like a certain area can be flabby or really show that you were heavier at one time. This is why I talked about an instructor, someone to help you along the way as you lose the weight in a good and proper manner. They may be able to help you figure out exactly where you want to be weight wise, what's suitable for your height, age, etc. This is in no way to promote any type of gym, aerobic center, work out place or anything of that nature. I only say this to you because I'm looking forward to you, the reader, writing me and telling me how well you have done and that you have met your weight loss goals. I can't encourage you to get there by taking this precious time trying to promote something else. It is essential that you are followed up by someone at some given time. You may just need their motivation, or their experience as a professional. So, making time for your workouts, exercises or whatever you do is very important to your weight loss. You also might want to gather your money up along the way to pay for these services, if you can afford it, pay all at one time so that the money won't be a hindrance to you when you want to attend their facility. Another way of doing things right is, when you have made so many mistakes with the same situation that someone else might be going through, it seems unconscionable to not tell the whole truth about things, and not to lead the people to believe that what they are doing is going to be a bed of roses. This is why I am sharing my blunders, as well as my success with you. There is no such thing as a victory without a fight. So, hopefully I am giving you enough ammunition to fight until you conquer your dragons and part of that ammunition is to inform you on how to do things right. When I didn't do things safely or I didn't do things wisely, I paid dearly every time. If it wasn't not doing this, it was not doing that, it seemed to be always something I had to put extended time out on, or extra money out on so I started learning to do it right from the beginning. The beginning for me was after I made what seemed like a thousand mistakes, then I looked back and kept seeing nothing but a mess. Then I finally said, wait, it seems like I've been here and done this before. It was then that I began to watch what I did and what I didn't do because these were the things that were going to cost me in the long run. I got wiser and wiser, not because I wanted to, but because I had to. I was losing money, time and effort. I had to catch on to this doing it right thing, or I was going to take 10 years to do this one thing, lose the weight. It behooved me to take a little more time with myself and with what I was doing. I needed to do things that would work out in my favor instead of work against me all the time. This was my big opportunity to turn this whole thing around and make me some lemonade. The kind of lemonade you can drink and say, that was a little bitter, but it was still good. That's what some of you, as the readers, might want to say. I may have made a mess of this weight loss thing, but it's time to make some lemonade. It's time to stop making blunders and to start doing things right because you don't want to spend any more time in your state than you have to. You want to be in a place where you can stop losing money by joining weight loss centers and never going or sacrificing to buy foods you need to complete your weight loss task, but still frying the chicken anyway. If you could just stop right in the middle of your tracks, and take a good hard look at yourself and watch your day to day activities you might change your mind about some things. Monitor whether you are doing things right, smart, or healthy because only you can answer that question. You are the one who knows if you have taken your medications properly while exercising or if you have been raiding the refrigerator at 3:00 in the morning, which you and I both know doesn't help your cause so think about yourself and figure out what is your best way to make sure that you do things right. Consider everything; your children, your career, your finances, your character, whether you like to get up early or go to bed late, so that you manage your schedule properly. A lot more goes into your losing the weight than getting on a treadmill or walking, or exercising every day. Hopefully reading this book, you have developed a mind to go on and win your prize but as you very well see, there is a price to pay, and you have to go into losing the weight with that frame of mind and be prepared for the booby traps, the disappointments, the messes, and whatever else that comes your way to oppose your weight loss. After you pay the price and make all your sacrifices as far as rest, time, entertainment, etc., whatever you have to curb to get to your weight loss goals, will definitely be worth it in the end. I dare not say that I am an expert on any of the things I spoke about in this book but I do say that I write from my experiences, failures, mistakes, downfalls and victories but most of all I have hopefully succeeded in persuading you to take care of yourself and to love yourself, and to not neglect the needs of your body. You can lose every ounce of weight you want to if you really try hard enough and put your mind to it. You can conquer the weight, don't continue to allow the weight to conquer you. There is only, always and forever going to be one of you, nobody else will ever know anybody like you. You are unique in your own very special way and you deserve to be happy and to enjoy life to the fullest. The way you want to enjoy it.

As I bring this book to a close, I'd certainly like to say that it has been a pleasure to serve you in this capacity. I sincerely hope that you have been encouraged to pursue your weight loss goals and have made up your mind that a change has to come about in your life and you are going to make things happen. Everything about you just might have to change, but only you can make it be for the good, if you set it up that way. As I said, be encouraged, and if you don't remember anything else I said, remember this; don't look back but look ahead because that's where things really matter. I hope you have enjoyed reading this book and I invite you to look for many more books in the future that will motivate, inspire and challenge everything in you to be the very best you can be.

Again, looking to hear from you, please find contact information on one of the following pages.

NOTES

_____

_____

_____

_____

_____

_____

_____

_____

_____

_____

_____

_____

_____

_____

NOTES

NOTES

NOTES

NOTES

www.ingramcontent.com/pod-product-compliance
Lightning Source LLC
Chambersburg PA
CBHW031303280526
45784CB00004B/1971